Mindreadings: literature and psychiatry

Edited by Femi Oyebode

RCPsych Publications

RCPsych Publications is an imprint of the Royal College of Psychiatrists, 17 Belgrave Square, London SW1X 8PG
http://www.rcpsych.ac.uk

British Library Cataloguing-in-Publication Data.
A catalogue record for this book is available from the British Library.
ISBN 978 1 904671 60 2

Distributed in North America by Publishers Storage and Shipping Corp.

The views presented in this book do not necessarily reflect those of the Royal College of Psychiatrists, and the publishers are not responsible for any error of omission or fact.

The Royal College of Psychiatrists is a charity registered in England and Wales (228636) and in Scotland (SC038369).

We have made every effort to contact the copyright holders of the poems included in this book. We thank those that have given their permission to include poems, in part or in full, and apologise to the few that we could not trace. If they would like to contact us, we will rectify attributional errors in any future reprint.

'Ill on a journey' by Basho, translated by T. Oseko in *Basho's Haiku: Literal Translations for Those Who Wish to Read the Japanese Text, with Grammatical Analysis and Explanatory Notes*, copyright © 1990 Chuoh Printing.

'Eleven addresses to the Lord' from *Collected Poems 1937–1971* by John Berryman, reproduced by permission of Faber and Faber Ltd.

'The asylum dance' from *Selected Poems* by John Burnside, published by Jonathan Cape. Reprinted by permission of The Random House Group.

'To God', 'An appeal for death' and 'The shame' from *Collected Poems* by Ivor Gurney (ed. P. J. Kavanagh), copyright © 1982 Carcanet Press.

'A mental hospital sitting-room', 'from Michelangelo's Sonnets', 'Night sister' and 'Sequence in hospital' from *New Collected Poems* by Elizabeth Jennings, copyright © 2002 Carcanet Press.

'War Music' from *War Music* by Christopher Logue, reproduced by permission of Faber and Faber Ltd.

'Home' and 'Visitors' from *Day by Day* by Robert Lowell, copyright © 1975 Farrar, Strauss and Giroux LLC.

'The addict', 'Clothes' and 'Wanting to die' by Anne Sexton. Reprinted by permission of SLL/Sterling Lord Listeric, Inc. Copyright © Anne Sexton.

'Not waving but drowning', 'Come, Death' and 'The hostage' by Stevie Smith, from *Collected Poems of Stevie Smith*. Reprinted by permission of New Directions Publishing Corps.
    USA, its territories and Canada: copyright © 1972 Stevie Smith.
    UK and rest of the world (excluding USA and Canada): copyright © 1972 Estate of James MacGibbon.

Printed by Bell & Bain Limited, Glasgow, UK.

Contents

Contributors

Allan Beveridge Consultant Psychiatrist, Queen Margaret Hospital, Dunfermline, UK

Gordon Bates Consultant in Child and Adolescent Psychiatry, Huntercombe Hospital, Stafford and Solihull Care Trust, Solihull, UK

Ed Day Senior Lecturer in Addiction Psychiatry, University of Birmingham, and Honorary Consultant in Addiction Psychiatry, Birmingham & Solihull Mental Health Foundation Trust, UK

H. M. Evans Principal, Trevelyan College; Professor of Humanities in Medicine, Centre for Medical Humanities, Durham University, UK

Anupama Iyer Consultant in Adolescent Developmental Psychiatry, St Andrews Hospital, Northampton, UK

Femi Oyebode Professor of Psychiatry, University of Birmingham, Birmingham, UK

John Skelton Professor of Clinical Communication, College of Medicine and Dentistry, University of Birmingham, UK

Iain Smith Consultant Psychiatrist and Honorary Clinical Senior Lecturer, University of Glasgow, Glasgow, UK

Christopher A. Vassilas Consultant in Old Age Psychiatry, Ashcroft Unit, Queen Elizabeth Psychiatric Hospital, Birmingham, UK, and Director of Medical Education, Birmingham and Solihull Foundation Mental Health Trust

Preface

Femi Oyebode

The emergence of the field of medical humanities in the past decade signals, perhaps, a change in the character of medicine. There are now journals of medical humanities published here in the UK, in Europe and across the Atlantic in the USA. It is also no longer rare to have poetry columns in leading medical scientific journals; the *British Journal of Psychiatry* has a 'poems by doctors' column and *Advances in Psychiatric Treatment* a column for poems by poets who have a history of psychiatric illness. Furthermore, there are medical humanities centres and undergraduate courses within medical schools and there is a medical humanities website. So what are the medical humanities? What possible benefit could they have for medicine and for doctors? And is there a special role for the humanities within psychiatry?

The medical humanities are described as including medical ethics, medical sociology, social history of medicine, and the application of literature and the arts in general to medicine. It has been argued that the medical humanities can complement medical science and technology through the contrasting perspectives of the arts and humanities either by 'softening' medicine or, more ambitiously, by shaping the nature, goals and knowledge base of medicine (Greaves & Evans, 2000). The goal here is to reintegrate the humanistic skills of recording and interpreting human narrative experience into the core of medical knowledge (Evans, 2001). More specifically, Scott (2000) has argued that the arts may stimulate a medical practitioner's insight into common and shared patterns of response to critical situations, or into unique and individual responses to crises, and may also enrich the language and thought of the medical practitioner. What is implicit in these arguments is that there is something about the scientific stance that detaches the medical practitioner from the subjective experience of patients and, this argument goes, the arts or the humanities can facilitate the re-engagement of the practitioner with the subjective world of the patient. I do not believe that there is much to disagree with here. It is a truism that modern medicine and its accompanying technology can treat people either as part organs or simply as material substances without any inhabiting animating self with goals and projects. This aspect of medicine is as damaging to the patient as it is to the practitioner.

The medical humanities project uses various methods to achieve its aims. One of these is to use texts to raise humanities issues. Jane Macnaughton (2000) has described such a method using a philosophy text, Plato's *Republic*, and others have described courses that use literary texts, including autobiographical and fictional narratives, to stimulate discussion and sharpen the imaginative capacity of students and medical practitioners. The overriding aim of these various methods is to reassert the importance of the patient's biography and self-hood into the medical discourse or space. As Evans (2001) puts it, 'literature and the representative arts engage the question of how the idea of the expressive transcends or transforms the merely descriptive – within, and about, the experience of medicine'.

From the foregoing it is self-evident that whatever benefits the medical humanities may have for the rest of medicine, they are equally relevant for psychiatry. All psychiatric disorders, perforce, are disorders of persons. The symptoms and signs of the conditions are played out in the lives of real people and it is impossible to separate out the locale of the condition as distinct from the person. What the arts and humanities can do for psychiatry is to reinforce the importance of the subjective. Our current diagnostic approaches emphasise the objectivity of symptoms and understate the importance of how these symptoms are experienced by persons, this despite the fact that the roots of clinical psychopathology lie in phenomenology. What literature can do (autobiographical narrative is particularly good at this) is to express the patient's distress and subjective, but no less real, understanding of this distress in the language of everyday life. In other words the psychiatrist can have access to the sheer humanity of the experience in other than technical language. In this way we as psychiatrists can deepen our own understanding of the nature of these conditions and acquire a more felicitous language both to engage our patients with and to assimilate the subjective reality of their conditions. Like every other skill, our moral imagination, that is, our empathy, needs to be exercised and tested and literature provides a safe way of doing this.

This book grew out of the series of articles on literature and psychiatry published in *Advances in Psychiatric Treatment*. Each article has been re-worked and there are new chapters written specifically for this book. The chapters cover a wide field. There are chapters on why doctors should read fiction; the place of literature in medical education; the role of autobiographical and fictional narratives; poetry; letters; death and dying; addictions; ageing and dementia; intellectual disability; and autism. These chapters explore the description and representation of mental states; the lived experience of distress; the character of psychiatry as a system; and the institutional practices of psychiatry. What unites these chapters is their reliance on language in all its communicative aspects, in particular in the form of literary texts, as sources and tools for furthering our understanding of our patients and their conditions.

In *Lady Chatterley's Lover*, Lawrence (1928) compared listening in on (overhearing) the private affairs of other people to the novel. He wrote 'Here lies the vast importance of the novel, properly handled. It can inform and lead into new places the flow of our sympathetic consciousness, and it can lead our sympathy away in recoil from things gone dead. Therefore the novel properly handled, can reveal the secret places of life: for it is in the passional secret places of life, above all, that the tide of sensitive awareness needs to ebb and flow, cleansing and freshening' (1994 reprint, p. 101). It is clear that Lawrence understood the link between the natural curiosity of eavesdropping on other people and the use of literature as a means of understanding the inner life of others as well as of ourselves. It is also true that Lawrence more than most writers particularly understood the role of the novel in exposing how people feel and behave, in exploring what motivates our most intimate acts and in using words to best describe the indefinable emotions that determine our goals and cloud our judgements. It is this role of literature in examining, clarifying and defining human emotions, behaviour and thoughts that the chapters in this book exemplify.

References

Evans, M. (2001) Medical humanities for postgraduates. In *Medical Humanities* (eds D. Kirklin & R. Richardson). Royal College of Physicians of London.

Greaves, D. & Evans, M. (2000) Medical humanities. *Journal of Medical Ethics*, **26**, 1–2.

Lawrence, D. H. (1928) *Lady Chatterley's Lover*. Reprinted 1994. Penguin Books.

Macnaughton, J. (2000) The humanities in medical education: context, outcomes and structures. *Journal of Medical Ethics*, **26**, 23–30.

Scott, P. A. (2000) The relationship between the arts and medicine. *Journal of Medical Ethics*, **26**, 3–8.

CHAPTER 1

The benefits of reading literature

Allan Beveridge

Does literature have anything to offer clinicians? Until recent decades the answer would have been self-evident: exposure to the humanities was held to deepen the understanding of suffering and confer wisdom on clinical practice. In fact there had long been a fruitful interaction between medicine and the arts. Many clinicians wrote essays, novels and poetry, and writers embraced medical themes. In the 18th century, Tobias Smollett, a Scottish doctor, achieved fame as a novelist with such books as *The Adventures of Roderick Random* (1748) and *The Expedition of Humphry Clinker* (1771). John Keats, the great English Romantic poet, was a qualified doctor, and Laurence Sterne made frequent references to medicine, health and sickness in *The Life and Opinions of Tristram Shandy, Gentleman* (1759–69).

The 19th and early-20th century saw such medical authors as Georg Buchner, Anton Chekhov, Arthur Conan Doyle, Mikhail Bulgakov, Arthur Schnitzler and William Carlos Williams. Even Emil Kraepelin, viewed by some historians of psychiatry as an incorrigible somaticist, was a published poet. The eminent French neurologist Jean-Martin Charcot dubbed the 'Napoleon of the Nerves', held evening soirees to which the leading writers, artists and doctors of Paris flocked. The great modernist writer Marcel Proust was influenced by many physicians and psychologists, including Binet, Charcot and Janet. His father was a professor of public hygiene and co-authored a book on nervousness. Proust's vast masterpiece *À la recherche du temps perdu (In Search of Lost Time)* (1913–27) deals with several medical and psychiatric topics, including hypochondria, hysteria, grief and mental breakdown (Micale, 2007).

Sigmund Freud was well versed in European and classical culture and his case reports were admired as much for their literary as for their scientific merits. In the second half of the 20th century, the Scottish psychiatrist R. D. Laing drew on writers such as William Blake, Dostoyevsky, Kafka, Beckett and Jean-Paul Sartre to construct his existential model of madness, and in the latter part of his career he also wrote poetry.

At some point, however, there appears to have been a loosening in the link between the arts and medicine. In an influential lecture, C. P. Snow, the physicist and writer, contended that society was divided into 'two cultures', the scientific and the artistic (Snow, 1959). He maintained that this split was destructive and warned that 'Closing the gap between our cultures is a necessity in the most abstract intellectual sense, as well as the most practical'. The origins of the rift between the arts and the sciences are often traced to the Enlightenment, which held that reason would solve the problems of humanity. The Romantic movement, which stressed spontaneity, the spiritual and a sense of wonder, is seen as hastening the division between the arts and the sciences.

However, this chronology has recently been challenged by the historian Mark Micale (2007), who argues that the relationship between the humanities and medicine continued to enjoy a mutually rewarding relationship until at least the early part of the 20th century. He maintains that the relationship began to falter only after the First World War with the ending of the liberal arts education to which doctors had previously been exposed. Rousseau (1986) has maintained that the value that clinicians attach to the humanities has waned in modern times and that doctors increasingly see themselves as scientists and biotechnicians. However, Neve (1993) has argued that, despite the prevailing technological culture, many doctors have maintained an interest in the arts.

In fact recent years have seen a resurgence of interest in the relationship between medicine and the arts. There has been the publication of the journal *Medical Humanities*; the rise of narrative-based medicine, with its insistence that reading literature can help doctors better understand the 'narratives' of their patients; and the creation of the Centre for Arts and Humanities in Health and Medicine at Durham University. Medical schools such as Glasgow and Birmingham now offer modules in the humanities. Such developments spring from the belief that it is beneficial for doctors to be exposed to the arts; that somehow it makes them better clinicians. This chapter will examine the benefits to psychiatrists of reading literature.

The benefits of reading literature

Existential aspects and empathy

A purely bioscientific model offers a limited view of human beings. Doctors need a deeper understanding of their patients that takes account of emotional and existential aspects. Literature offers such a perspective (Downie, 1994). The changes in medical education outlined in *Tomorrow's Doctors* (General Medical Council, 1993) recommended that students be exposed to the humanities as well as the biosciences. There is some evidence that medical students who have a background in the humanities and science, rather than science alone, go on to perform better in important areas of practice (Rolfe *et al*, 1995). In relation to psychiatry, Cawley (1993) has argued that medical science does not provide a complete picture of human beings and advocates the complementary study of the humanities.

T. S. Eliot (1948: p. 86) observed that 'we read many books, because we cannot know enough people'. We can explore the lives and inner worlds of a wide variety of individuals by imaginatively engaging with them in novels. One can see the world from another person's viewpoint. This is especially applicable to literary accounts of illness and suffering. For example, Iain Crichton Smith's novel *In the Middle of the Wood* (1987) depicts his own psychotic breakdown; Evelyn Waugh's *The Ordeal of Gilbert Pinfold* (1957) describes drug-induced hallucinosis; Bernard MacLaverty's *Grace Notes* (1997) deals with postnatal depression; Ian McEwan's *Enduring Love* (1997) is concerned with de Clérambault's syndrome; and practically all of Dostoyevsky's novels feature characters with mental disturbances. Such work helps us to develop empathy with people who suffer from mental illness.

Mental illness does not take place in isolation: it affects relatives and the wider society. Jacqueline Wilson, the award-winning children's author, demonstrates this to great effect in her novel *The Illustrated Mum* (1999). The book is concerned with a character called Marigold, who has bipolar disorder and who is also the mother of two girls. The story is told through the eyes of her 10-year-old daughter Dolphin, and it shows the impact of mental illness on a family. We see Dolphin's anxiety as her mother becomes unwell and her attempts to contain and deal with Marigold's increasingly wayward behaviour. We also see the tensions between Dolphin and her elder sister as they argue about how best to 'manage' their mother. In one scene, Dolphin describes what happens when her mother comes to pick her up from school and is obviously elevated in mood and somewhat disinhibited:

> I came out of school the next day and there was Marigold, waiting for me. She was standing near the other mothers but she stuck right out. Some of the kids in the playground were pointing at her. Even Owly Morris blinked through his bottle-glasses and stood transfixed.
>
> For a moment it was if I had borrowed his thick specs and was seeing her for the first time. I saw a red-haired woman in a halter top and shorts, her white skin vividly tattooed, designs on her arms, her shoulders, her thighs, one ankle, even foot.
>
> I knew several of the fathers had tattoos. One of the mothers had a tiny butterfly on her shoulder blade. But no-one had tattoos like Marigold.
>
> She was beautiful.
>
> She was bizarre.
>
> She didn't seem to notice that none of the mothers were talking to her. She jumped up and down, waving both hands when she saw me.
>
> 'Dol! Dolly, hi! Yoohoo!'
>
> Now they weren't just staring at Marigold. They were staring at me too.
>
> I felt as if I were on fire. I tried to smile at Marigold as I walked towards her. My lips got stuck on my teeth. I felt that I was wading through treacle.
>
> 'Dol, quick!' Marigold shouted.
>
> I got quicker because she was making so much noise [Wilson, 2000: pp. 46–47].

In this passage the reader identifies with Dolphin and shares her embarrassment and mounting sense of trepidation about her mother's behaviour.

In contrast to the more detached position of the psychiatrist assessing a patient, we are plunged into the everyday reality of life with a mentally ill relative. Alan Bennett has written poignantly about his mother's depressive illness and the effect it had on him and his family. He freely admits that he found her condition exasperating and that he was relieved that the main burden of care eventually fell on his father rather than him. In this extract Bennett describes his mother's condition and his reaction to it:

> The onset of depression would find her sitting on unaccustomed chairs – the cork stool in the bathroom, the hard chair in the hall that was just there for ornaments and where no one ever sat, its only occupant the occasional umbrella. She would perch in the passage, dumb with misery and apprehension, motioning me not to go into the empty living room because there was someone there.
> 'You won't tell anybody?' she whispered.
> 'Tell anybody what?'
> 'Tell them what I've done.'
> 'You haven't done anything.'
> 'But you won't tell them?'
> 'Mam!' I said exasperated, but she put her hand to my mouth, pointed at the living-room door and then wrote TALKING in wavering letters on a pad, mutely shaking her head [Bennett, 2005: p. 6].

Numerous people have written about their experiences of consulting psychiatrists (Porter, 1991). These accounts allow us to see the psychiatric encounter from the other side and should make us more aware of how our words and behaviour affect our patients. In *Mrs Dalloway* (1925), Virginia Woolf, who herself suffered from mental illness, portrays the psychiatrist as patronising, a view echoed in Janice Galloway's *The Trick is to Keep Breathing* (1989). In contrast, Iain Crichton Smith describes a helpful psychiatrist in his novel *In The Middle of the Wood* (1987). The American poet Sylvia Plath, who battled with depression, saw several psychiatrists and described her impressions of them – both the good and the bad – in her novel *The Bell Jar*. In the following passage we see how her fantasies of how a psychiatrist should behave clashed disappointedly with the reality.

> Doctor Gordon twiddled a silver pencil.
> 'Your mother tells me you are upset.'
> I curled in the cavernous leather chair and faced Doctor Gordon across an acre of highly polished desk.
> Doctor Gordon waited. He tapped his pencil – tap, tap, tap – across the neat green of his blotter.
> His eyelashes were so long and thick they looked artificial. Black plastic reeds fringing two green, glacial pools.
> Doctor Gordon's features were so perfect he was almost pretty.
> I hated him the minute I walked in through the door.
> I had imagined a kind, ugly, intuitive man looking up and saying 'Ah!' in an encouraging way, as if he could see something I couldn't, and then I would find words to tell him how I was so scared, as if I were being stuffed farther and farther into a black airless sack with no way out.

Then he would lean back in his chair and match the tips of his fingers together in a little steeple and tell me why I couldn't sleep and why I couldn't read and why I couldn't eat and why everything people did seemed so silly, because they only died in the end.

And then, I thought he would help me, step by step, to be myself again.

But Doctor Gordon wasn't like that at all. He was young and good-looking, and I could see right away he was conceited [Plath, 1966: pp. 135–136].

Aesthetics

The so-called 'aesthetic' approach to the medical study of literature is claimed to lead to the development of complex interpretive skills (McLellan & Jones, 1996). Narrative-based medicine is particularly concerned with this area (Greenhalgh & Hurwitz, 1998). The techniques involved in understanding and analysing a novel can be applied to the understanding of patient discourse. One can become more sensitive to the nuances and subtexts of a patient's communication.

Several literary devices have clinical resonances. For example, the concept of the 'unreliable narrator' is especially applicable to the understanding of a patient's history. This refers to the situation where the character telling the story gives, either by design or unwittingly, a misleading or distorted account of events. For example, in *The Diary of a Nobody* (1892) by George and Weedon Grossmith, the narrator Charles Pooter attempts to present himself as a man of dignity, but his account of himself and his encounters with others reveals that he is a figure of fun. The reader responds to the tale the narrator is telling with the feeling that there is another interpretation than the one being offered. For example, Pooter takes a great pride in his diary and has been in the habit of reading it to his wife and son. However, he records that it is 'disappointing to me … that Carrie and Lupin take no interest whatever in my diary'. He continues:

> I broached the subject at the breakfast table today. I said: 'I was in hopes that, if anything ever happened to me, the diary would be an endless source of pleasure to you both: to say nothing of the chance of the remuneration which may accrue from its being published.'
> Both Carrie and Lupin burst out laughing. Carrie was sorry for this, I could see, for she said: 'I didn't mean to be rude, dear Charlie; but truly I do not think your diary would sufficiently interest the public to be taken up by a publisher [Grossmith & Grossmith, 1995 reprint: p. 128].

Here we can see that Mr Pooter is deceiving himself that his diary is of interest and is publishable. His account of his family's reaction to the diary suggest to the reader that it is actually of no interest to anyone except himself. The reader is also alerted by Pooter's pompous prose that he is not quite the figure of his own estimation. A similar phenomenon can occur clinically when a patient's story suggests to the psychiatrist a very different picture than is intended. It may be the language the patient uses, or how they present their own character in the narrative that provides clues for the attentive listener.

Another literary device that has clinical relevance is where two or more narrators tell the same story. The reader then has to decide which version provides the most convincing interpretation of events. Does a particular narrator give a more accurate account? Does the 'truth' lie somewhere in between? Is no version reliable? Or is the notion of a single 'truth' untenable, as postmodernist thinkers contend? (Beveridge, 1998).

One of the first novels to confront the reader with different versions of the same event was *The Private Memoirs and Confessions of a Justified Sinner* (1824) by James Hogg. The novel has a narrative by the central character Robert Wringhim, who recounts how he has been possessed by an evil, satanic figure who has caused him to commit murderous crimes. There is another narrative by an 'editor' who attempts to give a 'rational' explanation of the extraordinary events described in the first narrative by maintaining that Wringhim is mentally ill. The reader has to decide whether to interpret the story as one of demonic possession or as one of insanity. Deliberately, Hogg does not privilege one interpretation over another.

This situation is familiar to the psychiatrist, who is often given different accounts of the same situation from the patient, the relatives, nurses and other doctors. The clinician then has to decide how much weight to give to each account. As in the novel, this is a process: as new information is presented the opinion of the doctor may change. Psychiatrists have to be aware of their own prejudices so that they do not automatically grant a particular witness more credibility. In Hogg's novel, for example, the medically minded reader may feel more disposed to favour the narrative of the editor, who seems to represent reason and rationality, and to view the account by Wrighim as the ravings of a madman. Hogg is careful to undermine this response and he shows that there are discrepancies and implausibilities in the editor's story too. Indeed, any narrative represents a particular, individual construction of events, and this needs to be borne in mind by the reader or psychiatrist.

Ethics

The 'ethical' approach to literature is said to lead clinicians to reflect on the moral implications of their practice. For example, Brian McCabe's story 'The full moon' (in *Selected Stories*, 2003) examines the feelings engendered in a therapist when he is mistaken for a patient. The therapist probably considers that he has a liberal and democratic approach to people with mental illness. However, as he is sitting in an art therapy session he is identified by a visiting psychologist as a psychiatric patient. His initial reaction is one of horror and he wants to declare that he is a member of staff and that he has a degree in philosophy. It is brought home to the reader that liberal sentiments may be superficial. We can make sympathetic noises about breaking down the barriers between 'them' and 'us' as long we are safely on the side of the barrier marked 'us'.

Literature can explore moral quandaries and how we arrive at clinical decisions. For example, William Carlos Williams' short story 'The use of force' (1938) raises the question as to whether medical intervention against a patient's will is ever justifiable. A paediatrician and a general practitioner, Williams was also a writer. In this short story he drew on his clinical experiences to depict a family doctor's encounter with a young child. When the doctor arrives at the family home he finds the parents anxiously waiting for him with their young daughter. He realises that the girl is very ill and may be suffering from diphtheria as there have been several recent cases at her school. The problem arises when he tries to examine her throat to confirm the diagnosis. The young girl is having none of it.

At first the doctor tries to win her confidence, using her first name and smiling in his 'best professional manner'. This does not work and we see how the situation unfolds. The parents try to help, but ineffectually. At one stage they say to their daughter, 'He won't hurt you.' The doctor is annoyed that they have used the word 'hurt', which he feels will only frighten the child more. The doctor for his part grows increasingly angry and it becomes for him a battle in which he must be triumphant.

We see that although the clinical situation presents a clear ethical dilemma – should force be used to examine the child's throat? – the doctor is making the decision in an emotionally charged atmosphere. He is agitated and the parents, embarrassed by the intransigence of their daughter, are urging the doctor to act.

After the child destroys the wooden tongue depressor with her teeth, the doctor makes a last attempt with a spoon. By this stage he has lost his 'reason':

> Get me a smooth-handled spoon of some sort, I told the mother. We're going through with this. The child's mouth was already bleeding. Her tongue was cut and she was screaming in wild hysterical shrieks. Perhaps I should have desisted and come back in an hour or more. No doubt it would have been better. But I have seen at least two children lying dead in bed of neglect in such cases, and feeling that I must get a diagnosis now or never I went at it again. But the worst of it was that I too had got beyond reason. I could have torn the child apart in my own fury and enjoyed it. It was a pleasure to attack her. My face was burning with it [Williams, 1984 reprint: p. 59].

Williams describes the feelings of the doctor as he tries to examine the child:

> The damned little brat must be protected against her own idiocy, one says to one's self at such times. Others must be protected against her. It is a social necessity. And all these things are true. But a blind fury, a feeling of adult shame, bred of a longing for muscular release are the operatives. One goes on to the end [pp. 59–60].

There is of course a good ethical case for trying to examine the young girl: she could easily die if nothing is done. Psychiatrists use the argument that they are acting to protect the patient from themselves when they treat an individual against their will, and often it is entirely justified. However, Williams shows how the personal feelings of the doctor can intrude into the decision-making. Ethical decisions are made in the messy and sometimes unsettling encounter between staff, patients and their relatives. This short story illustrates much more powerfully than a textbook on ethics the dilemmas that everyday clinical practice throws up and how the personalities of the participants influence the outcome.

There are countless other literary examples of ethical dilemmas. In *The Citadel* (1937) by A. J. Cronin, who was himself a doctor, the main character Dr Andrew Manson examines a patient whom he thinks is faking illness. Should the doctor sign the sickness certificate the patient wants, or should he confront the man? The first option is the one of least resistance, and the second is potentially acrimonious. Dr Manson chooses to confront his patient, who reacts in a threatening and abusive manner. Once again, we see that ethical decisions are made in the clinical setting and that they have consequences for doctor and patient alike.

It is worth pointing out that although the reader is expected to applaud the heroic actions of the doctor, Cronin's text unintentionally undermines this. He describes the patient in a highly judgemental way: he is 'a great lump of a man, rolling in fat, who smelled strongly of beer and looked as if he had never done a full day's work in his life' (1973 reprint: p. 108). The language employed by the author serves to remind us that our supposedly noblest actions may be based on contempt.

Additive and integrated approaches to literature

Commentators have discussed the difference between an 'additive' and an 'integrated' approach to reading literature (Evans & Greaves, 1999). The former sees the arts as adding to an existing bio-medical knowledge base, so that, for example, we might start from the traditional categories of psychiatric disease and seek out literary accounts that illustrate these conditions.

The 'integrative approach' attempts to refocus the whole of medicine to an understanding of what it is to be fully human. Richard Smith (1999) has observed, 'The additive view is that medicine can be 'softened' by exposing its practitioners to the humanities; the integrated view is more ambitious, aiming to shape the nature, goals and knowledge base itself'.

One of the earliest novels to question the role of medical science was *Frankenstein. Or the Modern Prometheus*, by Mary Shelley, which was first published in 1817. The story has of course entered popular mythology and people are more likely to be acquainted with it through film than by reading the book. Mary Shelley had a serious aim in writing *Frankenstein*: to examine the moral implications of scientific advances. Victor Frankenstein, a student of natural philosophy, chemistry and anatomy, strives to discover how to create life. Although he is successful, the creature he brings into being breaks free from his control and goes on to wreak havoc. Victor Frankenstein is guilty of hubris: of believing he is God. Readers are shown that progress in medicine may have unintended consequences and that there is always a moral dimension to it. Mikhail Bulgakov (1925) provided a humorous perspective on the Frankenstein story in *The Heart of the Dog*, in which a professor implants the testicles and pituitary gland of a human being into a stray dog. Again the procedure has unintended and unfortunate consequences as the newly formed creature goes on to cause mayhem in the professor's home. Georg Buchner, in his play 'Woyzeck' (1836, published posthumously 1879), depicted a doctor who experiments on a patient, with a fatal disregard for the moral implications of his research: as a result the patient is led to commit murder.

The 19th-century Russian writer Fyodor Dostoyevsky lived at a time when many people felt that science would ultimately solve all the questions of humanity. In our day there are some neuroscientists who claim that the problems of human beings will be explained entirely in terms of brain function. Dostoyevsky rejected this biological, reductionist view of mankind. His novel *Notes from the Underground* (1864) offers a critique of such notions. The central character observes ironically:

> science itself will teach man ... that he really has neither free will nor caprice and never did, and that he himself is nothing more than a kind of piano key or organ peg ... everything he does, he does not at all according to his wanting, but according to the laws of Nature. Consequently, one only has to discover these laws of Nature and then man will not answer for his acts ... All human actions, of course, will then be calculated by these laws, like a table of logarithms...
> [quoted in Thompson, 2002: p. 196].

Dostoyevsky felt that such theories deprived man of free will, and he rejected this materialist, biological psychology. Moral decisions depend on free choice, but if, as claimed by science, there is no free will, then there can be no morality. In *The Brothers Karamazov* (1880), Ivan Karamazov makes the famous observation that if this view was correct then 'everything is permitted'. Dostoyevsky thus challenges psychiatrists who take a narrowly biological approach to mental illness. He suggests that viewing human beings as mechanisms is not only misguided but that it has moral implications.

Of course, the question of applicability of the natural sciences to human beings has long been debated, for example in the so-called *methodenstreit* or methodological controversy in late-19th century. There were positivist thinkers such as John Stuart Mill, August Comte and Emile Durkheim, who argued that the natural scientific model is appropriate because humans are essentially no different from the rest of the physical world. Against this view were theorists such as Wilhelm Dilthey and Max Weber, who argued that humans are distinct as a result of possessing free will, consciousness and a need for meaning. Consequently, a different approach was necessary and they argued that the humanities, such as history and literature, have an important role in helping to understand people.

We see this debate continuing today, with some arguing that the humanities have nothing to offer doctors. For example, Wassersug (1987) has declared: 'real medical progress has not been made by humanitarians but by doctors equipped with microscopes, scalpels, dyes, catheters, rays, test tubes, and culture plates'. Similarly, there are those who feel that psychiatry should be seen as a branch of the natural sciences. Human beings are essentially no different from other constituents of the physical world, and all we need to know about them will be revealed by the neurosciences.

Another writer who was uneasy about the application of science to human problems was Aldous Huxley. In his 1932 novel *Brave New World*, he described a future that is organised and controlled by medical technology. At the 'Central London Hatchery and Conditioning Centre' human beings are created by genetic engineering and subsequently programmed by behavioural techniques. A rigidly hierarchical society is manufactured and its citizens are further controlled by a medication called soma. The heavy price to pay for this pharmaceutical and genetic-based social order is the loss of freedom. Individuals no longer have free will.

Huxley was not against science as such, but he was alarmed at the possibilities for its misuse and misapplication. In the foreword to his novel he contended that human beings should look within to spiritual factors, rather than without to technology to solve their problems.

There are contemporary resonances with Huxley's account of soma, an agent that keeps the citizens happy. One of the characters, Bernard Marx, who feels out of place in the utopian society, objects to the drug: ' "I'd rather be myself," he said. "Myself and nasty. Not somebody else, however jolly" '. His companion Lenina asks him: ' "Why you don't take soma when you have these dreadful ideas of yours. You'd forget all about them. And instead of feeling miserable, you'd be jolly. So jolly" ' (Huxley, 1977 reprint: pp. 75–76).

Huxley anticipates our own era, in which happiness is seen as a right. There has been a massive rise in the prescription of antidepressants (Healy, 1997) and the names of psychotropic medication have entered popular consciousness with, for example, Elizabeth Wurtzel entitling her novel *Prozac Nation* (1994). Self-help manuals abound, a situation that has been satirised by Will Fergusson in his book *Happiness*™ (2003). Huxley makes us question whether universal happiness – even if it is attainable – is such a good idea. Would it undermine what it is to be human? He also makes us question the role of pharmacology in society. Do drugs distort or even obliterate our personality?

Huxley highlights an issue that is important for psychiatrists, that of conformity. A popular perception of psychiatrists is that they are social policemen, patrolling society for any evidence of deviance from the norm. Psychiatrists, of course, have to decide what to make of apparently odd behaviour. Is it a sign of illness or is the person just unconventional? Huxley shows that a society in which everyone conforms is an immensely boring one. Another writer who has explored the question of conformity is Eugene Ionesco in *Rhinoceros* (1950). In this absurdist play, the characters, one by one, turn into rhinoceroses. One man, Berenger, tries to resist this trend and we see that he is left in a lonely and isolated position. It is easier to go with the herd.

Some objections to the notion that reading is beneficial

Not everybody agrees that reading literature makes for better doctors. Some contend that imaginative writers are attempting to do crudely and unsystematically what modern psychologists do in a sophisticated and rigorous manner. According to Downie & Charlton (1992) it is enough to state this proposition to recognise the absurdity of it, but there are those who agree with it. David Lodge dramatised the conflict between literature and psychology in his novel *Thinks* (2001), in which a cognitive scientist and a novelist argue over whether science or imaginative literature offers the best way of unlocking the mysteries of the mind. The cognitive scientist claims that imaginative literature is merely 'folk psychology'.

However, it is by no means proven that psychological concepts and terminology offer a more profound or revealing account of human beings. A work that examines the limitations of 'scientific' language is *The Memorandum* (1965), a play by the Czech writer Vaclav Havel. The play has analogies with the attempts in psychiatry and psychology to create a 'scientific' or 'technical' language to describe emotional and mental distress. Such language can lead to a dehumanising approach to the sufferer. R. D. Laing made this point nearly 50 years ago in *The Divided Self* (1960), when he looked at psychiatrists' attempts to provide 'objective' terminology for their patients' self-reports.

In *The Memorandum*, Havel takes an absurdist look at the endeavours of officialdom to introduce a more 'scientific' language. The authorities hope that the new language will 'make office communications more accurate'. The language is called Ptydepe, and according to one of its adherents:

> Ptydepe ... is a synthetic language, built on a strictly scientific basis. Its grammar is constructed with the maximum rationality, its vocabulary is unusually broad. It is a thoroughly exact language, capable of expressing with far greater precision than any current natural tongue minutest nuances ... the natural language originated, as we know, spontaneously, uncontrollably in other words, unscientifically, and their structure is thus, in a certain sense, dilettantish [Havel, 1993 reprint: pp. 65–66].

Havel shows the folly of such a venture. The Ptydepe language is cumbersome and unusable. Attempts to make rigid rules to control the spontaneity of human speech are doomed. A character called Josef Gross objects to the new language:

> ...every single member of the staff is human ... If we take from him his human language, created by the centuries-old tradition of national culture, we shall have prevented him from becoming fully human and plunge him straight into the jaws of self-alienation [p. 18].

Havel's examination of the uses and abuses of language has relevance to psychiatry. Attempts at developing 'technical' terms to describe a person's mental and emotional experience run the risk of turning the patient into an object. One does not necessarily have to subscribe to a conspiratorial view of psychiatry to acknowledge that the language psychiatrists use frames how they see their patients and as a consequence how they treat them. If psychiatrists talk about their patients as if they are objects, they are less likely to see them as autonomous individuals with their own point of view.

Harold Bloom (2000), a distinguished literary critic, asserts that reading does not make us better, more caring people. It is essentially a selfish activity. It can expand an individual's intellectual horizons but it does not engender altruism or increased sensitivity to others. In his book *Newton's Sleep*, the physician Raymond Tallis (1995) goes to great lengths to argue that an acquaintance with the arts does not make individuals more caring; in fact, it might make them less so. He quotes Tolstoy's tale of an aristocratic woman weeping in the theatre at the imaginary tragedy enacted on the stage, while outside a real tragedy is taking place as her faithful coachman freezes to death. Here art serves to deceive the woman that she is sensitive, when she is actually inconsiderate. More generally, George Steiner (1971) has repeatedly questioned the assumption that exposure to the arts leads to more civilised behaviour, citing the example of Nazi Germany, where high culture coexisted alongside concentration camps. As McManus (1995) has pointed out, the semantic kinship between the terms humane and the humanities suggests a causal relationship, but there may, in fact, be none.

Reading is not a substitute for experience. Marcel Proust, who immersed himself in literature, recognised this. As he wrote: 'To make [reading] into a discipline is to give too large a role to what is only an incitement. Reading is on the threshold of the spiritual life; it can introduce us to it: it does not constitute it' (Proust, quoted in de Botton, 1997: p. 197).

An exclusively bookish life can lead to an estrangement from the rest of humanity. In an amusing historical survey entitled 'Reading: a health warning', Roy Porter (1999) charted the many voices, including physicians and psychiatrists, who have advised that excessive reading can bring about mental and physical decline. From the artistic point of view, several commentators object to the whole notion of approaching a work of literature with the pre-determined aim of extracting something that may be clinically 'useful' (Bamforth, 2001). Imaginative writing should produce varied and unpredictable responses in its readers. It is inappropriate to trawl through literature for references to doctors and disease, as this implies that the reader is not open to the aesthetic potential of the work. Oscar Wilde famously declared, 'All art is quite useless', and resisted any suggestion that it is educational or morally uplifting.

Psychiatrists who read literature evidently see value in it; those who do not might be unmoved by arguments in its favour. Those who argue against the benefits of reading are surely right to question the assumption that exposure to literature automatically brings about greater sensitivity and empathy in the reader. However, there is a growing acknowledgement of the value of the humanities in medical education, and perhaps this is part of a wider trend that recognises the limitations of a purely biotechnological approach to patient care. In a critique of evidence-based medicine, Williams & Garner (2002) conclude that it 'must be underpinned by the need to understand and respond empathically to the illness in accord with the patient's experiential perspective', and they go on to underline the importance of engaging with the humanities as part of professional development.

If one does accept that it is of benefit to psychiatrists to read, should there be a canon of improving texts? Several such have indeed been pro-posed (Greenhalgh & Hurwitz, 1998; Bamforth, 2003). However, there is a danger that they are approached as didactic texts. Reading them can then become a chore. Furthermore, if the aim is to develop interpretive skills, it could be argued that it does not matter what books are read; they do not have to be about medicine, psychiatry or mental illness.

However, one of the claims in favour of reading is the notion that books about illness and suffering help doctors to better understand the inner experience of their patients and, as a consequence, to develop greater empathy. It is here that a suggested reading list may be of value. It is important that such lists are offered in the spirit of suggestion rather than as compulsory texts. It will then be left to the individual psychiatrist to decide whether they are worth exploring. A medical culture that takes a positive approach to the humanities will greatly encourage such explorations.

References

Bamforth, I. (2001) Literature, medicine, and the culture wars. *Lancet*, **358**, 1361–1364.

Bamforth, I. (2003) *The Body in the Library. A Literary Anthology of Modern Medicine*. Verso.

Bennett, A. (2005) *Untold Stories*. Faber & Faber.

Beveridge, A. (1998) The detective, the psychiatrist and postmodernism. *Psychiatric Bulletin*, **22**, 573–574.

Bloom, H. (2000) *How to Read and Why*. Fourth Estate.

Cawley, R. H. (1993) Psychiatry is more than a science. *British Journal of Psychiatry*, **162**, 154–160.

Cronin, A. J. (1937) *The Citadel*. Reprinted 1973. New English Library.

de Botton, A. (1997) *How Proust Can Change Your Life*. Picador.

Downie, R. S. (1994) *The Healing Arts*. Oxford University Press.

Downie, R. S. & Charlton, B. (1992) *The Making of a Doctor. Medical Education in Theory and Practice*. Oxford University Press.

Eliot, T. S. (1948) *Notes Towards the Definition of Culture*. Faber & Faber.

BEVERIDGE

Evans, M. & Greaves, D. (1999) Exploring the medical humanities. *BMJ*, **319**, 1216.

General Medical Council (1993) *Tomorrow's Doctors*. General Medical Council.

Greenhalgh, T. & Hurwitz, B. (1998) *Narrative Based Medicine*. BMJ Books.

Grossmith, G. & Grossmith, W. (1892) *The Diary of a Nobody*. Reprinted 1995. Penguin.

Havel, V. (1965) *Vyrozumení*. Reprinted (1993) as *The Memorandum* in *The Garden Party and Other Plays*. Grove Press.

Healey, D. (1997) *The Antidepressant Era*. Harvard University Press.

Huxley, A. (1932) *Brave New World*. Reprinted 1977. Panther Books.

McLellan, M. F. & Jones, A. H. (1996) Why literature and medicine? *Lancet*, **348**, 109–111.

McManus, I. C. (1995) Humanity and the medical humanities. *Lancet*, **346**, 1143–1145.

Micale, M. (2007) Two cultures revisited: the case of the fin de siècle. In *Medicine, Madness and Social History. Essays in Honour of Roy Porter* (eds R. Bivins & J.V. Pickstone), pp. 210–223. Palgrave.

Neve, M. (1993) Medicine and literature. In *Companion Encyclopedia of the History of Medicine* (eds W. F. Bynum & R. Porter), vol. 2, pp. 1520–1535. Routledge.

Plath, S. (1966) *The Bell Jar*. Faber & Faber.

Porter, R. (1991) *The Faber Book of Madness*. Faber & Faber.

Porter, R. (1999) Reading: a health warning. In *Medicine, Mortality and the Book Trade* (eds R. Myers & M. Harris), pp. 131–152. St Paul's Bibliographies.

Rolfe, I. E., Pearson, S., Powis, D. A., *et al* (1995) Time for a review of admission to medical school? *Lancet*, **346**, 1329–1333.

Rousseau, G. S. (1986) Literature and medicine: towards a simultaneity of theory and practice. *Literature and Medicine*, **5**, 152–181.

Smith, R. (1999) Editor's choice – struggling towards coherence. *BMJ*, **319**, 0a.

Snow, C. P. (1959) *The Two Cultures and the Scientific Revolution*. Cambridge University Press.

Steiner, G. (1971) *In Bluebeard's Castle: Some Notes towards the Re-definition of Culture*. Faber & Faber.

Tallis, R. (1995) *Newton's Sleep. The Two Cultures and the Two Kingdoms*. Macmillan Press.

Thompson, D. O. (2002) Dostoyevsky and science. In *The Cambridge Companion to Dostoyevsky* (ed. W. J. Leatherbarrow), pp. 191–211. Cambridge University Press.

Wassersug, J. D. (1987) Teach humanities to doctors? Says who? *Postgraduate Medicine*, **82**, 317–318.

Williams, W. C. (1938) The use of force. In *Life along the Passaic River*. Reprinted (1984) in *The Doctor Stories*. New Direction Books.

Williams, D. D. R. & Garner, J. (2002) The case against 'the evidence': a different perspective on evidence-based medicine. *British Journal of Psychiatry*, **180**, 8–12.

Wilson, J. (1999) *The Illustrated Mum*. Reprinted 2000. Corgi Books.

CHAPTER 2

Roles for literature in medical education

Martyn Evans

'Do you see it, young man?' This is how the *Hofrat* (medical director) of the tuberculosis sanatorium situated on the slopes of Thomas Mann's *Magic Mountain* (1927) invites Herr Hans Castorp, the book's flawed young hero, to gaze into the primitive fluoroscope image of his ailing cousin Joachim:

> And to the pulsation of the floor, and the snapping and cracking of the forces at play, Hans Castorp peered through the lighted window, peered into Joachim Ziemssen's empty skeleton. The breastbone and spine fell together in a single dark column. The frontal structure of the ribs was cut across by the paler structure of the back. Above, the collar-bones branched off on both sides, and the framework of the shoulder, with the joint and the beginning of Joachim's arm, showed sharp and bare through the soft envelope of flesh...
>
> ...But Hans Castorp's attention was taken up by something like a bag, a strange, animal shape, darkly visible behind the middle column, or more on the right side of it – the spectator's right. It expanded and contracted regularly, a little after the fashion of a swimming jellyfish.
>
> 'Look at his heart,' and the Hofrat lifted his huge hand again from his thigh and pointed with his forefinger at the pulsating shadow. Good God, it was the heart, it was Joachim's honour-loving heart that Hans Castorp saw! [1996 reprint: p. 127].

Set in the years leading up to the outbreak of the First World War, and written only a little later than the period in which it was set, this is effectively a contemporary account of the early appearance in the medical armoury of imaging technology – here, the fluoroscope – and the astounding impact it must have made on the layman encountering it for the first time. A 'witches' kitchen' is how Mann describes the whole imaging laboratory, complete with a 'private thunderstorm' of electrical discharges and glowing retorts.

Of historical interest, perhaps; but not only that. The teller of tales makes the tale come alive. Consider the shock and excitement of discovery – not only in a Wellsian technological past but right here and right now – of making the invisible become visible, of 'anatomising' the interior of a still-living body, a body just like your own in every important respect. Sometimes a carefully articulated image is used: he peered through the *lighted window,* he peered into Joachim Ziemssen's *empty skeleton*. Sometimes the sparest of prose is enough: *Good God, it was the heart!* The reader who has sat with Hans Castorp through his journey and arrival at the sanatorium – who has sat with him at the interminable meals and despaired of his artless efforts to impose youthful originality and independence on suffocating bourgeois conversation – who has frequently wanted to strangle him and half the sanatorium's inhabitants – the reader who, in short, after 200 pages has stumbled upon the chapter called 'Sudden enlightenment' and feels himself sorely in need of it, now walks alongside Castorp, trembling, through the arched doors of Mann's arch prose into the Gothic vaults of the X-ray chamber; and now the reader steps, head spinning, up to the fluoroscope machine itself as if it were tomorrow's lurid prophesy and not yesterday's medical commonplace. But much, much more:

> A few minutes later [Hans Castorp] himself stood in the pillory, in the midst of the electrical storm, while Joachim, *his body closed up again*, put on his clothes. Again the Hofrat peered into the milky glass, this time into Hans Castorp's own inside; and from his half-utterances, his broken phrases and bursts of scolding, the young man gathered that what he saw corresponded to his expectations. He was so kind as to permit the patient, at his request, to look at his own hand through the screen. And Hans Castorp saw precisely what he must have expected, but what it is hardly permitted man to see, and what he thought it would never be vouchsafed him to see: *he looked into his own grave.* The process of decay was forestalled by the powers of the light-ray, *the flesh in which he walked* disintegrated, annihilated, dissolved in vacant mist, and there within it was the finely turned skeleton of his own hand, the seal ring he had inherited from his grandfather hanging loose and black on the joint of his ring-finger – a hard, material object with which man adorns the body that is fated to melt away beneath it, when it passes on to another flesh that can wear it for yet a little while … [With] penetrating, prophetic eyes, he gazed at this familiar part of his own body, *and for the first time in his life he understood that he would die* [pp. 218–219, my italics].

A passage like this either leaves you coldly unmoved or it stops your heart. To those left unmoved, I am afraid I probably have nothing interesting to say (unless it be to direct you elsewhere in this book). But if for you, as for me, the ideas in this passage are as electrifying as the processes generating the vision of Hans's grave, and if for you this prose – even in the stilted English of the earliest published translation from the German – is itself a form of radiant, albeit spooky, illumination, then I will try to suggest how (and why) that illumination might be harnessed within medical education and the making of doctors, psychiatrists among them.

Four medical educational 'goods' – and literature's support for them

Let us take it as read that medical education must instil and refine the medical student's scientific understanding of how the human body works – of how it contracts, develops, resists, overcomes or succumbs to disease at the physiological and anatomical levels. I want my doctor to know all of this – and if necessary all of *me* – inside out. But let me suggest both how this can be built upon or augmented, and also how it can be subverted.

These days, the augmentation is actually pretty commonplace: namely, that clinical skills and competencies involve the ability to find out what is wrong with me, by examining me both physically *and personally*. By examining me 'personally', I mean here discovering and understanding what is individual about me, and how my individuality is necessary to treating me. These abilities are variously referred to as communication skills, narrative skills, skills of interpretation, interpersonal skills, ethical awareness and so on, and it seems sensible to suppose that a good (albeit guided) soaking in decent literature might offer anyone who wants it an opportunity to enrich the abilities they already possess.

In this context, McLellan observes that the skills of literary interpretation of texts help doctors consider 'the totality of the lives of patients they may meet only in limited, fragmented ways' (McLellan, 1996: p. 110). Again, Charon tells us that the study of literary methods 'help[s] doctors and patients to achieve *contextual* understandings of *singular* human experiences' and that such study supports 'the recognition of multiple contradictory meanings of complex events' (Charon *et al*, 1996: p. 243, my italics).

Such capabilities obviously augment the biomedical knowledge expected of the doctor, but I think they can be seen in some ways as subverting that knowledge. This might seem like an overstatement, but medicine is part of the human endeavour of healing, and ought to be conceived in that light. Humans are not machines, and the ways in which we fall ill and our prospects for getting better are intensely influenced by the 'existential' questions, challenges and events in our lives. So 'examining me personally' (as distinct from examining me physically) is not simply a way of being efficient, speedy and courteous in getting at the somehow purely scientific information the doctor needs. 'Examining me personally' is the necessary way of getting the complete range of information relevant to the diagnosis, and not all of that information is well captured by biomedical science.

'Examining me personally' means finding out something of the salient facts of my 'case' as that 'case' feels to me – the person who lives the life in question. Why do I do what I do? Why are my ambitions and vulnerabilities what they are, and how do they bear on my tendency to get sick or stressed-out or flabby or dependent on an additional glass or two of wine – in the manner that is particular to me? Is my self-esteem appropriate and healthy? How do I see myself, my work, my relationships – do they inspire me or corrode me? And so on. And these are not determinate facts – by which I mean that they do not correspond to a tick in a box, or a block on a chart. They are perceptions – either held by me, or held about me by others and responded to by me. They are *inter*-personal, and in gathering some idea of them, the clinician enters an interpersonal connection with me in which her own perceptions become influential. Worse still, they are variables which are shockingly resistant to being controlled, and hence resistant to being understood or explored – still less experimented on – within a biomedical model as ordinarily pictured. Whether, of course, we should allow the ordinary model of science to escape lightly with no acknowledgement of the personal and interpersonal dimensions of even simple experimental observation is another matter (Polanyi, 1958; Toulmin, 1993).

As I have elsewhere expressed it, the lives, experiences and understandings of the doctor and the patient can be thought of as two tracks across a world that is not by any means fully mapped out. Where those tracks cross, their different pasts and futures shape the way each understands the other. Their different understandings naturally supply and fix the images and metaphors each will use. Most intriguingly, the clinical encounter is a meeting of two uniquely embodied experiences, each of which has somehow to make sense of and respond to the other (Evans, 2002). Not only medical science, but also literature and history and philosophy and anthropology and psychology (among others) are at stake in understanding and describing that encounter.

Clinical medicine is both practically and (to my mind, as a layman) theoretically inseparable from the sorts of considerations that – when studied systematically – you would find in the disciplines of literature, history, ethics, philosophy, psychology and so forth. Properly understood, clinical medicine is an intervention in what might be called the *existential* world as well as in the natural world (Toulmin, 1993). I am frequently struck by the thought that some of the most remarkable features about our embodied human condition can be caught by acknowledging our carnal nature – the fact that we are *meat* – but also by then recognising (as the phenomenologist philosophers have long urged that we recognise) that our carnal nature is the ground and the form of our conscious experience and our understanding of ourselves – the fact, that is, that we are *meat with a point of view* (Evans, 2002).

Far more of our nature and situation is intensely physical than we are inclined to remember. I fear I am putting this point rather drily, as philosophers tend to do. It will be more real – as well as being more succulent – if I let the experience of one of classic literature's great characters, Konstantin Levin, put the point for me. Here, in a glowing passage from *Anna Karenina* (1876), Tolstoy describes Levin's unconscious sense of his own physicality and well-being as it emerges from the unaccustomed experience of mowing the ripe hay in the fields that he owns, but which he has hitherto never mown in the way that his peasant tenants mow them:

> In the very heat of the day, the mowing did not seem such hard work. The perspiration with which he was drenched cooled him, while the sun, that burned his back, his head and his arms bare to the elbow, gave a vigour and dogged energy to his labour; and more and more often now came those moments of oblivion, when it was possible not to think of what one was doing. The scythe cut of itself. Those were happy moments. Still more delightful were

the moments when they reached the river at the end of the rows and the old man would rub his scythe with a thick knot of wet grass, rinse the steel blade in the fresh water of the stream, ladle out a little in a tin dipper, and offer Levin a drink.

'What do you say to my home-brew, eh? Good, eh?" he would say with a wink.

And truly Levin had never tasted any drink so good as this warm water with bits of grass floating in it and a rusty flavour from the tin dipper. And immediately after this came the blissful, slow saunter, with his hand on the scythe, during which he could wipe away the streaming sweat, fill his lungs with air, and look about at the long line of mowers and at what was happening around in the forest and the country.

The longer Levin mowed, the oftener he experienced those moments of oblivion when it was not his arms which swung the scythe but the scythe seemed to mow of itself, a body full of life and consciousness of its own, and as though by magic, without a thought being given to it, the work did itself regularly and carefully [1954 reprint: p. 273].

Our sense of ourselves, our appearance, our capacities, our immediate movements, our place, our relations to others, the extent to which we are at ease in a given situation, our awareness of our surroundings, our expectations of what will happen to or around us in the next moment, our hopes, our plans, our hearts' desires, our terrors and dismay – all of these have an intensely physical basis that it is often convenient to us to suppress or forget: but I think we are philosophically and psychologically and, indeed, clinically mistaken when we do so. And curiously – perhaps because in our paper-driven word-bound world we are rarely allowed so primarily physical an experience of ourselves and our surroundings as that enjoyed by Kostya Levin – we are usually much better at remembering our physical nature when we are sick than when we are well. So clinical medicine is deeply driven by, and aims at modifying, our experiences of ourselves in sick or disabled or distressed states. It aims at intervening in our nature in order to relieve those experiences; it aims at an intervention in *the point of view* as well as in the meat. Clinical medicine inevitably has historical, philosophical, social, psychological and of course intensely literary dimensions, and these ways of looking at the people who present as patients are, I think, inescapably part of the clinical encounter – whether or not they are formally prepared for, or even recognised or acknowledged, by clinicians themselves.

There are practical and, in a sense, moral objections to this enlarged picture of the clinical encounter, of course. Here, rehearsed very briefly, are five such objections.[1] The personal and interpersonal aspects of the encounter may be what some patients fear or resent above all others; we ought not to assume that every patient is willing to be 'examined personally' any more than we can simply assume permission for a physical examination. Even granted such

---

1 I am grateful to Heidi Lyth for pointing out to me the five objections here.

permission, we cannot know in advance what will be disclosed or what will be its implications: the clinical encounter may not be the best place to acknowledge the chaotic and destructive nature of some people's lives, although perhaps psychiatry above other specialties steels itself to attempt that task. In the face of this, there is a sense of comfort, for the general clinician, in the retreat to a narrow physiological paradigm: from within its protection, the clinician can apparently more fairly ask of the patient: 'Just what is it you want from me?', and more reasonably refuse to offer, through *medicine*, any 'existential' guarantees about the patient's life and prospects. Simply preparing for medicine's personal dimension seems arduous – an enlarged specification for medicine seems only to add to the educational hurdles over which the unfortunate student must leap. Moreover, the personal dimensions of the clinical encounter are true for the clinician as well, whose embodied, carnal experience from time to time includes exhaustion, frustration and (in the ordinary sense) depression.

I am not going to address these objections directly, other than to acknowledge their force while yet insisting that they really show that clinical medicine's inevitably personal dimension is a tough, albeit rewarding, challenge for which medical education must do more to prepare tomorrow's doctors. My starting point is that the larger question of what medical knowledge actually *is* must finally be considered in these humanistic terms as well as in the more familiar scientific terms (Toulmin, 1993). So, therefore, is the deeply connected question of how that knowledge is to be gained. This then invites us to consider a wider range of medical educational 'goods' than simply the bio-scientific understanding of the body's physiological workings.

What might these other 'goods' be? Allow me to suggest the following four, of which the first three are either explicit or implicit in the General Medical Council's landmark publication *Tomorrow's Doctors* (General Medical Council, 1993).

Education, not training

First, there is the emphasis on education as distinct from training, and education moreover in an appropriately university-based medical curriculum. This perhaps requires a little elaboration. Certainly, this 'good' is not exclusive to medicine: quite the reverse, as *Tomorrow's Doctors* implicitly complained. Medical schools have consistently recruited very high-achieving school leavers, then processed them through an intensely demanding, even exhausting, scheme of study. But a scheme of study that involves the assimilation of a gigantic number of facts is unlikely to be – and traditionally has not been – a rewarding challenge to the creative intellect. Education is, among other things, an invitation to step through doors into larger 'rooms', conceived in imaginative, cultural, intellectual and (to use a risky word) spiritual terms – an invitation to step into those rooms, look around, and above all appraise *for yourself* what you find in them. This should form part of the study experience of any mature professional who will be engaged in a sophisticated interpersonal practice. It should be the cornerstone of developing the clinical professional's own personal resources for dealing with the uncertainties, even the chaos, of the demands of clinical life and the attitudes, behaviours, needs and goals of patients. A role in this for the study of literature is, I hope, readily apparent. Education consists in an enlargement of vision, and this enlarged vision is well served by the accomplishments of literary interpretation identified by Charon *et al* (1996) and McLellan (1996).

Ethics and communication skills

The second educational 'good', and one which is perhaps rather more directly 'applied' to the clinical situation than was the first, is the development of medical students' communication skills, including (obviously) a sensitive appreciation of the ethical dimensions of their practice. As an intrinsically good thing, this second 'good' needs no further explanation. It also seems straightforward to suppose that the structured and studied interpretation of literary texts supports it, particularly in the terms Charon *et al* (1996) commend.

An objection sometimes raised in this context is that it is disreputable to 'use' literature (or, for that matter, any of the creative or expressive arts) in such an instrumental way – the arts should be pursued for their own sake, and not for the sake of what they can do for us (Pickering, 1998). I have some sympathy with this admittedly rather purist objection: it might be that, like humility, a capacity for sensitive interpretation is not something you can coldly and intentionally *go out and get*, although it might easily be the natural result of doing something else, namely approaching literary texts in the right spirit of seriousness and curiosity, and moreover doing so for their own sake. It is interesting that this objection seems not to apply to the study of other supposedly 'visiting' disciplines within the medical curriculum (such as psychology or philosophy or history) and reflects, I think, a special intimacy with which we engage literature and the – as it were – tender place we accord literature that we love.

The answer to the objection, in my view, lies in how we choose, present and explore the texts themselves: Mann's *The Magic Mountain* or Kafka's *The Metamorphosis* (1915) are good examples of daunting texts that one might approach 'instrumentally', with anxiety and distaste, only to embrace them with passion and leave them tenderly: loving them for their own sake, perhaps not even noticing – until the time comes when it will really count – that one's awareness of the complexity and ethical sensitivity of situations and contexts is richer than it was.

21

Developing personal values

The third 'good' is that of encouraging students to identify, explore, develop and sustain their own personal values. It is not always easy to say exactly what we believe in or what our values are, even from the imagined vantage point of middle age and mid-career. How many of us in that position entirely recall the values we suppose ourselves to have held as youthful idealists, at the outset of our careers or our university degree courses? Did we graduate with a well-formed set of personal values – or did they accrete around us, accidentally, unplanned, as part of our *ad hoc* responses to the crises (personal or professional) that came our way? The traditional medical curriculum may have presumed some traditional professional values, but the habits of loyalty and the closing of ranks do not constitute a complete set of ethics, nor need they come naturally and authentically to every clinical practitioner facing the occasional clash of interests between patient and professional, or patient and institution. Such situations perhaps can never be properly prepared for – authentic moral life, I suspect, can never consist in *complete* preparation, but must always allow room for spontaneous reaction to the particularities of precisely this or that situation. Even so, it is better to have thought about what you believe in before you put your beliefs to the test, and it seems to me that this is one of the attitudes and facilities that we should try to develop in students of all disciplines: why not students of medicine, tomorrow's front-line clinical practitioners? And where better than in the comparative safety of the literary encounter to test, and extend, your range of beliefs and attitudes? As the *Oxford Handbook of Clinical Specialties* (Collier *et al*, 1995: p. 413) puts it:

> When we read alone and for pleasure, our defences are down – and we hide nothing from the great characters of fiction. In our consulting rooms, and on the ward, we so often do our best to hide everything, beneath the white coat, or the avuncular bedside manner. So often, a professional detachment is all that is left after all those years inured to the foibles, fallacies and frictions of our patients' tragic lives. It is at the point where art and medicine collide, that doctors can re-attach themselves to the human race and re-feel those emotions which motivate or terrify our patients ... *[E]very* contact with patients has an ethical and artistic dimension, as well as a technical one.

A sense of wonder

Fourth and finally, I suggest an educational 'good' that is not in fact implicit in *Tomorrow's Doctors*, but whose importance I think is implicit in the clinical encounter. It is not at all easy to express it: I would summarise it as the stimulation and encouragement of a fitting and enduring *sense of wonder* at embodied human nature. Let me try to say what I think this sense of wonder is or involves, and then say why it is important. The general idea of a sense of wonder is closely tied to curiosity, indeed, is probably the basis of some of our most important curiosity, driving the early investigations of the natural world and, I trust, the individual investigations carried on by many in science today. A sense of wonder is more than curiosity alone, however; it implies a kind of recognition of something's having special significance or even grandeur, so the recognition may sometimes amount to an attitude of awe or reverence. As such, a sense of wonder prompts reflective considerations about the place of mankind in the natural world and questions about whether 'the natural' is the sum total of the world, questions about what or who controls that world and about our individual destinies within it. Again, it would be hard to doubt that a sense of wonder has played a role in creative artistic responses to the world around us.

To approach something in wonder is to put yourself aside to some extent, to magnify the significance of the observed in relation to you who observe. The psychological importance of this is felt, for instance, when as a parent you contemplate your child; but also when you are struck by how experiences that you recognise in yourself belong also to other people – who, perhaps, respond to them as you would yourself like to respond (creatively, bravely, calmly, with insight) though you fear that in fact you could not. In this way, wonder is an important attitude ethically, reminding us that things, or people, or interests beyond ourselves are connected to us, but also have a claim on us – sometimes a higher claim than the mundane ones that normally see us through the working day. Literature peerlessly opens our eyes to wonder. I think the electrifying passage from *The Magic Mountain* with which I began exemplifies this perfectly, laying open to our gaze not only the literal but also the metaphorical wonder of our own physicality (*Good God, it was the heart!... He looked into his own grave... the flesh in which he walked [was] disintegrated, annihilated, dissolved in vacant mist*) in stunning yet sobering verbal apparitions.

Why is this clinically important? Those latter, ethical aspects are probably clearest, and apply quite straightforwardly to the praiseworthy list of 'attitudinal objectives' urged in *Tomorrow's Doctors*. To wonder at the fortitude of patients is, among other things, also to respect those patients. But a sense of wonder also invites us to incorporate gentleness, discretion, dignity and respect into that scientific curiosity which it is natural to feel towards so perplexing a phenomenon as the embodied, experiencing, human organism – who is also the patient. A lively and cultivated sense of wonder extends our capacity to be committed professionally to each successive individual, each particularised case of otherwise abstract and general disease categories and, moreover, stimulates a richly alert awareness of the diagnostic and therapeutic importance of easily missed variations in presentation and context. Above all, a sense of wonder – wonder at this wondrous intersection, fusion, of 'meat' and 'point of view' – is the bedrock of recognising the medical privilege of intervening in frail human flesh and experience. Being aware of that privilege could brighten the darkest of clinical days in the course of a demanding career.

References

Charon, R., Brody, H., Clark, M. W., *et al* (1996) Literature and ethical medicine: five cases from common practice. *Journal of Medicine and Philosophy*, **21**, 243–265.

Collier, J. A. B., Longmore, J. M. & Hodgetts, T. J. (1995) Fame, fortune, medicine and art. In *The Oxford Handbook of Clinical Specialties* (4th edn) (eds J. A. B. Collier, J. M. Longmore & T. J. Hodgetts), p. 413. Oxford University Press.

Evans, M. (2002) Reflections on the humanities in medical education. *Medical Education*, **36**, 506–507.

General Medical Council (1993) *Tomorrow's Doctors: Recommendations on Undergraduate Medical Education*. General Medical Council.

Mann, T. (1927) *Der Zauberberg*. Reprinted (1996) as *The Magic Mountain* (trans. H. Lowe-Porter). Vintage Books.

McLellan, F. (1996) Why literature and medicine? *Lancet*, **348**, 109–111.

Pickering, N. (1998) Imaginary restrictions. *Journal of Medical Ethics*, **24**, 171–175.

Polanyi, M. (1958) *Personal Knowledge: Towards a Post-critical Philosophy*. University of Chicago Press.

Tolstoy, L. (1876) *Anna Karenina*. Reprinted (1954): trans. R. Edmonds. Penguin.

Toulmin, S. (1993) Knowledge and art in the practice of medicine: clinical judgement and historical reconstruction. In *Science, Technology and the Art of Medicine* (eds C. Delkeskamp-Hayes & M. A. Gardell Cutter), pp. 231–249. Kluwer Academic Publishers.

CHAPTER 3

Autobiographical narrative and psychiatry

Femi Oyebode

Since St Augustine of Hippo's *Confessions*, written between AD 397 and AD 398, autobiographies have come to combine self-analysis and honest personal disclosure. It is therefore not surprising that there are auto-biographical accounts of mental illness, for honest self-disclosure has cachet only when the material that is disclosed is taboo. Thus, the *Confessions* was a remarkable work because it dealt with the saint's previous life of sin, especially his sexual weaknesses. However, it would be wrong to imply that autobiographical accounts of mental illness have all been written merely to be revelatory. There are accounts, such as J. S. Mill's *Autobiography* of 1873 and Janet Frame's three-volume work, published individually between 1983 and 1985 and as a trilogy (*An Autobiography*) in 1989, that set the author's experience of the illness in the context of a life, so that the account of mental illness sits appropriately within the trajectory of an existence that has other purposes and goals. There are other accounts, such as Fiona Shaw's *Out of Me* (1997) and Tim Lott's *The Scent of Dried Roses* (1996), which are as much about the experience of mental illness as the attempt to make sense of that experience. There are also accounts, such as Lewis Wolpert's *Malignant Sadness* (1999), that are examples of public health education of a refined kind. Sarah Ferguson's *A Guard Within* (1973) is distinct, in that it is epistolary in nature and is addressed to her deceased psychiatrist.

Autobiographical narratives of mental illness are unique sources of information. They allow psychiatrists and other mental health workers a rare insight into the richness of psychopathology as experienced, rather than as drawn out and described by psychiatrists. Furthermore, the impact of psychiatric illness and the consequences of being 'labelled' on the identity and social life of individuals can be more forcefully described. The variety of folk understanding, what is now technically termed health belief, is also revealed and given validity such that it challenges the perspective of psychiatry. The many rituals of psychiatry, the pernicious and restricting environment of hospitals and the importance of personal relationships with clinicians are all exposed and discussed in autobiographical narratives. It is evident that psychiatrists would benefit from reading them. They also offer an opportunity to become familiar, in a safe and unthreatening manner, with what our patients think of us and the services we provide. Books, at least, can be read in privacy. The emotionally charged views of many of our patients can be confronted without the impulse to become defensive. However, not all autobiographical accounts are critical of psychiatry or psychiatrists. And those that are also deserve to be read and understood.

The aim of this chapter is to examine the main themes found in auto-biographical narratives. For this purpose, I have excluded autobiographical novels such as Janet Frame's *Faces in the Water* (1961). I have also excluded fictional works, such as Patrick McGrath's *Spider* (1990), that treat mental illness or asylums as major issues. Journals and poetry have also been excluded. My choice of books is not exhaustive. There is an established tradition of borrowing from autobiographical narratives of mental illness. Jaspers, in his *General Psychopathology* (1913), borrowed from Schreber's *Memoirs of My Nervous Illness* (1903). Indeed, Freud (1911) and Sass (1994) have based their own notions of delusions on Schreber's *Memoirs*. In many respects, all psychiatrists owe a debt to Schreber, whose writing has helped to illuminate psychopathology and shape our understanding of psychotic experiences. This fact further underlines the importance of autobiographical narratives to psychiatry.

Psychopathology

Mood disturbance

Writers as diverse as J. S. Mill and Tim Lott describe their experience of mood disturbance with exceptional clarity. Mill's description of anhedonia, which appears in his *Autobiography* of 1873, stands out:

> It was the autumn of 1826. I was in a dull state of nerves, such as everybody is occasionally liable to; unsusceptible to enjoyment or pleasurable excitement; one of these moods when what is pleasure at other times, becomes insipid or indifferent ... In this frame of mind it occurred to me to put the question directly to myself, 'suppose that all your objects in life were realised; that all the changes in institutions and opinions which you are looking forward to, could be completely effected at this very instant: would this be a great joy and happiness to you?' And an irrepressible self-consciousness distinctly answered, 'No!' At this my heart sank within me [1989 reprint: p. 112].

Mill's intention in his autobiography was not to write about mental illness; thus he did not dwell for long on this aspect of his life. Neither did he understate or minimise his experiences. We are aware of the recurrence, severity and impact of his depressive episodes. We see that he considered suicide, but there is no melodrama in the account. We are left with the impression of an active intelligence, a generous spirit who is totally committed to human progress. His childhood and prodigious talent, his extraordinary erudition and accomplishments put his experience of depression into context.

In contrast to Mill's description of loss of enjoyment, we have William Styron's evocation of the anguish of depression: 'I was feeling in my mind a sensation close to, but indescribably different from actual pain' (1990: p. 16). This analogy between depression and physical pain recurs in many writers. Writing in 1902, William James described depression as follows: 'It is a positive and active anguish, a sort of psychical neuralgia wholly unknown to normal life' (1999 reprint: p. 165). For others, the intangibility of the emotional pain drives the individual to inflict actual physical harm that will result in real, that is, physical pain. For example, Sarah Ferguson (1973: p. 136):

> I slashed my wrist again and again, as deeply as I could. I knew perfectly well that it would not kill me, not like the times before … As my writing to you comes to a close, the pain is so unbearable inside me that a force of such strength has driven me to inflict a physical pain on myself in the hope of appeasing the other.

The intangibility of the experience of depression is described by Styron (1990: p. 7):

> Depression is a disorder of mood, so mysteriously painful and elusive in the way it becomes known to the self – to the mediating intellect – as to verge close to being beyond description. It thus remains nearly incomprehensible to those who have not experienced it in its extreme mode.

Styron continues:

> [I]t was past 4 o'clock and my brain had begun to endure its familiar siege: panic and dislocation, and a sense that my thought processes were being engulfed by a toxic and unnameable tide that obliterated any enjoyable response to the living world [p. 16].

> The pain of severe depression is quite unimaginable to those who have not suffered it, and it kills in many instances because its anguish can no longer be borne [p. 33].

> That fall, as the disorder gradually took full possession of my system, I began to conceive that my mind itself was like one of those outmoded small-town telephone exchanges, being gradually inundated by flood waters. One by one, the normal circuits began to drain, causing some of the functions of the body and nearly all of those of the instinct and intellect to slowly disconnect [p. 47].

It is easy to forget that depression, the mood disorder, is not merely a disturbance of emotional life, which it clearly is, but also a singular perturbation in the experience of one's own body, and of the world. Fiona Shaw's description of the effect of depression on how she experienced her body is worthy of note because it touches on an aspect of depression that is not remarked on in standard textbooks: 'My body became inert, heavy and burdensome. Every gesture was hard. … My existence was pared away almost to nothing, except for the self-contempt that bruised my eye sockets and throat, that turned my stomach and made my tongue into some large, coarse creature in my mouth' (Shaw, 1997: pp. 26, 27).

Then there are the recognisable effects on sleep, appetite, energy and enthusiasm:

> Sleep deserted me. And, no longer able to stomach myself, I stopped eating. There was no revulsion but I didn't want to eat anything [Jamison, 1995: p. 28].

> Depression is like an amoeba, altering its shape to take in every corner of my life; just when you think its left one place, it turns up in another. What is it that makes me, compels me, not to eat when I know I must? [Shaw, 1997: p. 30].

> Each day I awoke deeply tired, a feeling as foreign to my natural self as being bored or indifferent to life. Those were next. Then a gray, bleak preoccupation with death, dying, decaying, that everybody was born to die, best to die now and save the pain while waiting [Jamison, 1995: p. 38].

The relationship of depression to the loss of faith and hope is ever present in these narratives. There is also the inevitability of suicide. The pervasive, obtrusive and inescapable reality of suicide is under-appreciated by clinicians. Styron (1990: p. 52) described how 'many of the artefacts of my house had become potential devices for my own destruction; the attic rafters (and an outside maple or two) a means to hang myself, the garage a place to inhale carbon monoxide, the bathtub a vessel to receive the flow from my open arteries'.

Jamison, in her book *An Unquiet Mind*, described how, once she had decided to end her life, she 'was cold-bloodedly determined not to give any indication of my plans or the state of my mind. I was successful. The only note made by my psychiatrist on the day before I attempted suicide was: *Severely depressed. Very quiet*' (Jamison, 1995: p. 113).

This efficient and detached approach to suicide is echoed in Clifford Beers' book *A Mind that Found Itself* (1907). Beers, like Styron, described how suicidal thinking compels the individual to consider various methods that may be used. In Beers' case, he chose jumping from a height – and survived. His deliberate deception of his parents and relatives as to his intentions is instructive to psychiatrists. Once he had decided on a method, he distracted his parents' attention from the severity of his condition by behaving as normally as possible. The compulsive nature of suicidal thinking and the tendency to deceive others once the decision to make an attempt has been reached should be more widely understood by all clinicians but perhaps more so by the nurses who have charge of patients on a day-to-day basis. And of course, survival of an attempt is often accompanied not by relief but by disappointment:

> I took the thirty sodium amytal which I had been keeping ... My heart stopped beating, but they put me in a respirator, and attached me to a cardiac machine in an intensive care unit. Afterwards, I thanked them, but I did not mean it [Ferguson, 1973: p. 138].

Although it is true that feelings of hopelessness and desperation abound, and that suicidal thoughts can be ever present, there is also ambivalence. The desire to die is not always thoroughgoing and irresistible. It can be matched by an equal desire to stay alive: 'I couldn't escape the awful confines of my leaden body and downcast eye. I didn't want to live, but I couldn't bear to die' (Shaw, 1997: p. 40).

Depression is only one pole of the possibility of disturbed mood. Its counterpart is mania. Jamison (1995: p. 67) described the experience of manic elation very well and also the transition from joyful elation to dysphoric elation:

> When you're high it's tremendous. The ideas and feelings are fast and frequent like shooting stars and you follow them until you find better and brighter ones. Shyness goes; the right words and gestures are suddenly there, the power to captivate others a felt certainty. There are interests found in uninteresting people. Sensuality is pervasive and desire to seduce and be seduced irresistible ... But somewhere this changes ... Everything previously moving with the grain is now against – you are irritable, angry, frightened, uncontrollable, and enmeshed in the blackest caves of the mind.

Jamison's description of her illness is instructive. She is an academic psychologist with expertise in mood disorders. Her understanding of the biological origins, clinical features and treatments of bipolar mood disorder is that of an expert. This renders her biographical account especially illuminating. She is able to adopt the dual perspective of objectivity and subjectivity:

> I did not wake up one morning to find myself mad. Life should be so simple. Rather, I gradually became aware that my life and mind were going at an ever faster and faster clip until finally, over the course of my first summer on the faculty, they both had spun wildly and absolutely out of control. But the acceleration from quick to chaos was a slow and beautifully seductive one [p. 68].

> My memories of the garden party were that I had had a fabulous, bubbly, seductive, assured time. My psychiatrist, however, in talking with me about it much later, recollected it very differently. I was, he said, dressed in a remarkably provocative way, totally unlike the conservative manner in which he had seen me dressed over the preceding year. I had on much more makeup than usual and seemed to him, to be frenetic and far too talkative. He says he remembers having thought to himself, Kay looks manic. I on the other hand, had thought I was splendid [p. 71].

> There was a neuronal pileup on the highways of my brain, and the more I tried to slow down my thinking the more I became aware that I couldn't. My enthusiasms were going into overdrive as well ... [p. 72].

> When I am high I couldn't worry about money if I tried ... What with credit cards and bank accounts there is little beyond reach. So I bought twelve snakebite kits, with a sense of urgency and importance. I bought precious stones, elegant and unnecessary furniture, three watches within an hour of one another (in the Rolex rather than Timex class; tastes bubble to the surface, are the surface, in mania), and totally inappropriate sirenlike clothes [p. 74].

> Slowly the darkness began to weave its way into my mind, and before long I was hopelessly out of control. I could not follow the path of my own thoughts. Sentences flew around in my head and fragmented first into phrases and then words; finally only sounds remained [p. 79].

Jamison's description captures the thrill and energy that is mania. But in the end, she succumbs to psychosis: 'Not only had my thoughts spun wild, they had turned into an awful phantasmagoria, an apt but terrifying vision of an entire life and mind out of control. I screamed again and again. Slowly the hallucination receded' (p. 80).

Psychoses

There is a dearth of good descriptions of psychotic experiences compared with descriptions of mood disturbance. This difference is perhaps understandable given the effects of schizophrenia on motivation, drive and use of language. Nevertheless, John Perceval (1838), Schreber (1903) and Beers (1907) give outstanding descriptions of their psychotic experience. It is not the purpose of this chapter to discuss the clinical diagnoses of these authors but rather to use their writings to illustrate some aspects of psychotic experience. Both Schreber and Beers described what is now termed delusional misidentification syndrome. The example below is from Beers' (1907) autobiography:

> I soon jumped to a second conclusion, namely, that this was no brother of mine at all. He instantly appeared in the light of a sinister double, acting as a detective. After that I refused to speak to him again, and this repudiation I extended to all relatives, friends and acquaintances. If the man I had accepted as my brother was spurious, so was everybody ... For more than two years I was without relatives or friends, in fact, without a world, except that one created by my own mind from the chaos that reigned within it ... [p. 23].

> Though they all appeared as they used to, I was able to detect some slight difference in look or gesture or in intonation of voice, and this was enough to confirm my belief that they were impersonators, engaged in conspiracy, not merely to entrap me, but to incriminate those whom they impersonated [p. 52].

Schreber (1903) writes

> The few patients besides myself who sometimes appeared in the garden, all gave a more or less bizarre impression; in one of them I once thought I recognised a relative of mine, the husband of one of my nieces [1955 reprint: p. 96].

> In an attendant apparently employed for my special supervision I thought I recognised, perhaps because of accidental likeness, the attendant of the County Court who used to bring the files to my home during my six weeks of professional activity in Dresden [p. 104].

> I could understand such likeness occurring in two or three instances but not the fact that, as I will show, *almost all the patients in the asylum*, that is to say at least several dozen human beings, looked like persons who had been more or less close to me in my life [p. 104].

Schreber's *Memoirs* are instructive in many respects. Here we have an educated man from an illustrious family who is a senior judge writing of his experience of mental illness. His is a superior intelligence describing and commenting on his experiences. He analyses psychiatric conceptions of psychopathology, drawing on the literature of his day:

> By hallucinations one understands, a far as I know, stimulation of nerves by which a person with a nervous illness believes he has impressions of events in his external world, usually perceived through the sense of seeing or hearing, which in reality do not exist. Science seems to deny any reality background for hallucinations, judging from what I have read for instance in Kraepelin's *Psychiatry*, Vol. 1, p. 102 ff. 6th edition. In my opinion this is definitely erroneous, at least if so generalised [p. 223].

Schreber described a multitude of hallucinatory and passivity experiences. What is remarkable is the degree to which he retains a self-observant consciousness. He informs us that:

> For almost 7 years – except during sleep – *I have never had a single moment in which I did not hear voices.* They accompany me to every place and at all times; they continue to sound even when I am in conversation with other people, they persist undeterred even when I concentrate on other things [p. 225].

> One day – *in bright daylight* – I saw from my window directly in front of the walls of the building where I lived, a magnificent portico arise, just as if the whole building were going to be transformed into a fairy palace; later the image vanished [p. 107].

He gives numerous descriptions of passivity experiences, including made feelings, made acts and made vital events such as defecation:

> No change in these conditions occurred until the end of 1894 or early 1895. It coincided with another miraculous phenomenon, the *'cursed creation of a false feeling'*; ... such an influence by miracles on one's mood is *possible* as I have learned by experience, but I am unable to say more as to how it comes about [p. 129].

> I may say that hardly a single limb or organ in my body escaped being temporarily damaged by miracles, nor a single muscle being pulled by miracles, either moving or paralysing it according to the respective purpose [p. 131].

> All my *muscles* were (and still are) the object of miracles for the purpose of preventing all movements and every occupation I am about to undertake. For instance attempts are made to paralyse my fingers when I play the piano or write [p. 136].

> My *eyes* and the *muscles of the lids* which serve to open and close them were an almost uninterrupted target for the miracles ... attempts were made to close my eyes against my will, so as to rob me of visual impressions [p. 136].

> My fingers are paralysed, the direction of my gaze is changed in order to prevent my finding the right keys, my fingers are diverted on to the wrong keys, the tempo is quickened by making the muscles of my fingers move prematurely [p. 144].

> In my own person the advent of the bellowing-miracle when my muscles serving the process of respiration are set in motion by the lower God (Ariman) in such a way that I am forced to emit bellow noises, unless I try hard to suppress them; sometimes this recurs so frequently that it becomes almost unbearable and at night makes it impossible to remain in bed [p. 165].

Like everything else in my body, the need to empty myself is also called forth by miracles; this is done by forcing the faeces in the bowel forwards (sometimes also backwards) and when owing to previous evacuation there is insufficient material present, the small remnants in the bowel are smeared on my backside [p. 177].

A miracle simultaneously affects the *direction of my gaze* ... my eye-muscles are therefore influenced to move in a certain direction so that my glance *must* fall on things just created [p. 186].

One will in any case not dispute that I must *know myself* whether my eyes are *pulled* towards an indifferent object or whether I look at something interesting around me *of my own will* [p. 187].

What is remarkable about Schreber is his capacity to examine and reflect on his experiences, to be able to see how they deviate from normal day-to-day experiences, yet to conclude that they are real and do not point towards mental illness:

From the medical specialist's report I notice with some satisfaction that he himself attributes a certain *reality* to my hallucinations, in so far as he apparently does not doubt that the "voices" described in my Memoirs are in fact perceived by me. The *only* difference of opinion then is whether the subjective sensation of hearing voices is caused only by pathological functioning of my nerves or whether some external cause acts on them [p. 294].

Whatever people may think of my "delusions", they will sooner or later have to acknowledge that they are not dealing with a lunatic in the ordinary sense [p. 214].

John Perceval's narrative is as instructive as Schreber's. In Perceval we have the son of Spencer Perceval, the British Prime Minister, who was assassinated in 1812 in the House of Commons. John Perceval was admitted to the asylum run by Dr Fox at Brisslington near Bristol in January 1831, where he remained until May 1832 when he was moved to the asylum run by Mr Newington at Ticehurst in Sussex. He remained here until 1834. His book *A Narrative of the Experience of a Gentleman during a State of Mental Derangement to Explain the Causes and the Nature of Insanity, and to Expose the Injudicious Conduct Pursued towards Many Sufferers under that Calamity* was published in 1838 and the second volume in 1840. Perceval's description of his symptoms and of his treatment at the two asylums is detailed and illuminating. His account of the physical condition of the asylums and the situation of his fellow patients is illustrative of the state of the treatment of mentally ill people in England at the beginning of the 19th century. Like Schreber he had a lively intelligence, an analytic mind and a desire to understand the nature of his experiences.

Perceval's definition of what it is to have mental capacity, drawn as it is from his understanding of what it was like not to be fit to run his affairs, should still command our attention today:

A man who knows who and what he is, his position in the world, and what the persons and things are around him; who judges according to known, or intelligible rules; and who, if he has singular ideas or singular habits, can give a reason for his opinions and his conduct; a man who, however wrong he may act, is not misled by any uncontrollable impulse or passion; who does not idly squander his means; who knows the legal consequences of his actions; who can distinguish between unseemly and seemly behaviour, who feels that which is proper and that which is improper to utter, according to the circumstances in which he is placed; and who reverences the subject and the ministers of religion; a man who, if he cannot always regulate his thoughts and his temper and his actions, is not continually in the extremes, and if he errs, errs as much from benevolence and hesitation, as from passion and excitement, and more frequently: lastly, a man who can receive reproof, and acknowledge when he has needed correction [1962 reprint: p. 314].

In reaching this conclusion, Perceval gradually came to a realisation of the nature of his delusions and hallucinations. This process is itself remarkable given that it was unaided by effective treatment. The manner of his self-realisation sheds some light on how insight influences a person's reaction to psychotic experience:

> I suspect that many of the delusions which I laboured under, and which insane persons labour under, consist in their mistaking a figurative or a poetic form of speech for a literal one... [p. 270].

> If anyone knew how painful the task of self-examination and of self-control was, to which I devoted myself at that time, every minute without respite, except when I was asleep, in order that I might behave, and with the sincere desire of behaving becomingly; they would understand how cruel I felt it afterwards, when I required my liberty for the further pursuit of health and of strength of mind, to have it denied to me for fear of my doing any person any bodily harm [p. 271].

> Thus you will hear one lunatic declare that he is made of iron, and that nothing can break him; another that he is a china vessel, and that he runs in danger of being destroyed every minute. The meaning of the spirit is, that this man is strong as iron, the other frail as an earthen vessel; but the lunatic takes the literal sense, and his imagination not being under his control, he in a manner feels it [p. 271].

> I had observed at Brisslington that the thunder, the bellowing of cattle, the sounds of a bell, and other noises conveyed to me threats, or sentences of exhortation, and the like: but I had till now looked upon all these things as marvellous, and I had been afraid to examine into them ... I discovered, and I think very nearly in the manner I have stated above, the nature of this delusion; and prosecuting my examinations still further, I found that the breathing of my nostrils also, particularly when I was agitated, had been and was clothed with words and sentences. I then closed my ears with my fingers, and I found that if I did not hear words – at least I heard a disagreeable singing or humming in the ears – and that those sounds, which were often used to convey distinct words and sentences, and which at other times seemed to the fancy like the earnest cries, or confused debating, or expostulations of many spirits, still remained audible; from which I concluded that they were really produced in the head or brain, though they appeared high in the air, or perhaps in the cornice of the ceiling of the room; and I recognised that all the voices I had heard *in* me, had been produced by the action of the pulses, or muscles, or humours, &c. in the body – and that in like manner all the voices I had been made to fancy outside of me, were either formed from or upon different casual sounds around me; or from and upon these internal sounds [pp. 294–295].

33

The rituals of psychiatry

William Seabrook's *Asylum* (1935) was written simply to describe his experience of treatment for alcohol misuse in an American asylum in the early 1930s. As he says, 'I am not a reformer of public opinion or a propagandist. I am an adventure writer of sorts, and I write this mainly as the story of a strange adventure in a strange place' (p. 12). Seabrook documents hospital rules on admission: patients were showered and weighed; all property, including watch and clothing, was taken away; patients had to sleep with the doors left open and the lights were left on; and the day began at 6 a.m. He noted that:

> They have a holy terror of suicide or attempted, since straightjackets, muffs, and handcuffs have been thrown into the dustbin. – It always keeps them on their toes. It was a month before they would even let me have my wristwatch [p. 32].

> It was a strange world in which I was still a neophyte. It had its rituals – psychiatry sometimes seems crazier than any of the patients it treats. For instance, the ritual at the dances had to be experienced to be believed at all, and then you wondered how anybody could have invented it [p. 49].

In contrast, Clifford Beers' *A Mind that Found Itself* (1907) is a campaigning book. His cataloguing of the instruments of restraint and their effect on the patient deserves to be read. These instruments included straightjackets, camisoles, muffs, straps and mittens. The use of the muff to restrain the patient at night, while the single attendant sleeps, and also as a means of discipline on 'account of supposed disobedience', gives an insight into the physically coercive environment in which psychiatry was practised. He describes the use of seclusion:

> Acting on the order of the doctor in charge, one of them stripped me of my outer garments; and, clad in nothing but underclothes, I was thrust into a cell. Few, if any, prisons in this country contain worse holes than this cell proved to be. It was one of five, situated in a short corridor adjoining the main ward. It was about 6 feet wide by 10 long and of a good height … The walls and floor were bare, and there was no furniture. A patient confined here must lie on the floor [p. 124].

Beers described how the brutalising environment coarsened the sensitivity of newly appointed young attendants such that, soon after being appointed, they became as harsh as the others. Furthermore, he described how the harsh and violent environment made him more hostile and violent:

> Deprived of my clothes, of sufficient food, of warmth, of all sane companionship and of my liberty, I told those in authority that so long as they should continue to treat me as the vilest of criminals, I should do my best to complete the illusion [p. 146].

He argued that more fundamental than technical reform, cure or prevention was the need for a changed spiritual attitude towards the insane. Beers succeeded in describing the perverse structures and oppressive regime of the early-20th-century American psychiatric system. This was not far off Perceval's description of early-19th-century England:

> My right arm was fastened by a short chain to the wall and the strap pressed rather tightly across my chest, it was still something to have one arm free even in the straight waistcoat, and not to be galled by the fastening of the other [1962 reprint: p. 95].

> There are a few humane hearts that will shudder and the view of this position, recollecting my birth, my education, my talents, and that I had not been an impious or irreflecting man. But they will say it was the fault of the doctor, and though they condemn the doctor, still it was but the doctor. But no, oh! No, my elder brother came to visit me at this very time. I might almost say that he seemed guided by providence to detect the cruel infamies of my situation ... he saw me and took leave of me ... and he left me to my fate. So great, so rooted are this world's hypocrisies, so deep and wide spreading its duplicity! [p. 96].

It is easy to be self-congratulatory, particularly because of the absence of physical restraints and overtly punitive regimes in modern psychiatric hospitals. However, our wards are still permeated and characterised by a lack of respect for patients; a subtly coercive atmosphere still presides. It is true, too, that an unreflective and inhumane indifference to anguish can still be observed, a benign not malign neglect, yet neglect it most definitely is. The situation is complicated by a worsening intolerance by the public and undue emphasis by the political class and media on risk rather than care and compassion. Beers and Perceval both, sadly, are still relevant today.

Relationship with doctors

Sarah Ferguson's *A Guard Within* (1973) is written in the style of a letter to her deceased psychiatrist. It is illustrative of intense grief. It reminds us of the power of the therapeutic encounter. Even though the relationship that we witness was born and nurtured within a psychotherapeutic relationship, it is a signpost to the nature of the relationship that patients have with their doctors. Ferguson's writing shows how real this very unreal and special relationship is to patients. It illustrates the dangers of crossing the boundaries between the abstract fantasy world in which psychotherapy trades and the crude reality of the mundane exchange within the here and now. This is not the place to discuss the moral and technical dimensions of Ferguson's relationship with her therapist but her writing provides insight into the rarely expressed thoughts and feelings that patients have for their doctors:

> I always dressed up for you and hoped you would not know [p. 13].

> I felt your hands upon me. You held me firmly in your hands. You had never touched me before, and it made me snap like a branch into two, and I began to trust you to put me together [p. 17].

> One day, after many troubles, you were holding me, and my head was just touching your face, and I became stronger than you, and you became mine ...

my head was only just touching your face. We never spoke of it … I tell you, it became easier to be with you then (but not noticeably so), and my trust in you grew, that is all [p. 31].

So much of what we talked of can never be written. It was born and grew and developed but not visibly. There was no theatre. What was, remains within, and will never leave for it has become part of me. There are great regions in what I write to you that must be unexpressed … There must be areas of silence. It has to be [p. 85].

If our relationship had been exposed to a crowd, it would have been damaged; not broken, because] it was strong and unbreakable … Only under our own terms could it grow. It might have perished under a public glare because it was so real and true. There was no pretence [p. 120].

The book is particularly tragic because we know that in the end the author does not survive; that she kills herself. We also know that the death of her therapist has inserted brute reality into the therapeutic space and it is impossible not to wonder whether this fact on its own is not responsible for her death; that her suicide was not inevitable, that it was connected to the importuned death of her therapist.

The third volume of Janet Frame's trilogy *An Autobiography* is entitled *The Envoy from Mirror City* and describes her relationship with Dr Cawley at the Maudsley Hospital, London. The chapter entitled 'Dr Cawley and the luxury of time' describes her introduction to the doctor and explains why she took to him readily:

I think I was able to accept Dr Cawley because I was aware that his view was wider, over a range of studies and disciplines and personal experience, just as I had readily accepted Dr Miller because I knew he was interested in music and art. The qualifications of medicine and psychiatry were extensions of these men, not starting and ending points [Frame, 1990 reprint: p. 383].

I was also pleased to discover that Dr Cawley, like myself, was interested in the Here and Now and not in theories about the past, and our talks were largely at first an accounting process, an examination of my emotional, personal, and even financial budget … [p. 383].

I now had confidence in Dr Cawley, for I had not only seen myself developing and growing in his care, I had observed his own development as an assured psychiatrist who, I felt, would always respect the human spirit before the practice, the fashions and demands of psychiatry. I was influenced also by the persistence of Dr Cawley in being 'himself' and not some 'image' of a psychiatrist: he did not patronise or pretend … [p. 385].

It is obvious that our patients have views about us, about our personality, our attitudes and our approach to psychiatry. It is too easy to forget that, just as we appraise the patient, we too are being appraised, assessed and judged. The therapeutic encounter is two-way. This realisation should make it less likely that patients will come to feel like Fiona Shaw (1997) did:

And yes, do talk about yourself, it's a good idea. It soon became clear, however, that Dr A didn't intend me to talk to *her*. Her reputation was based principally 'upon her skill as a prescriber of medication' [p. 42].

Impact of diagnosis and labelling on social life

Janet Frame's autobiography (1983–85) describes her experiences of in-stitutional psychiatry in New Zealand and Britain and the lasting impact of these experiences on her. In both this work and her autobiographical novel *Faces in the Water* (1961) we learn how an individual can come to be processed through the psychiatric system and how the system, with its varied rituals, can strip an individual of identity and the sense of agency. The labels we use, no matter how valid, can have a force above and beyond clinical utility. It is as if the act of naming itself carries prognostications, like a shaman's pronouncement, both magical and social, that can imperil the patient's life. Frame wrote: 'I suffered from *schizophrenia*. It seemed to spell my doom, as if I had emerged from a chrysalis, the natural human state, into another kind of creature. ... I was taking my new status seriously. If the world of the mad were the world where I now officially belonged (lifelong disease, no cure, no hope), then I would use it to survive, I would excel in it' (*An Autobiography*, 1980 reprint: pp. 196, 198). This new status had social implications: 'I was in hiding. I was grieving. I didn't want anyone to "see", for once I had been in hospital, I had found that people didn't only "see", they *searched* carefully' (p. 211).

Frame helps us to see how, once labelled and treated as mentally ill, a person can become 'other', separated spiritually and socially from family and society. A sense of loneliness, of not belonging and of constantly being under scrutiny ensues and undermines confidence. This can result in the patient readily seeking asylum in the company of people designated as mentally ill, despite the fact that the asylum is neither welcoming nor a healthy refuge. Frame also helps us to see that a self-imposed restraint exists. Lack of confidence, shame and fearfulness combine to entrench a person further in misery. Part of this process is mediated by where the asylum is sited, the distinction drawn by the separation of the realm of the insane and the domain of the sane, and the response of family to the diagnosis of insanity:

> More trees appeared as the train approached Seacliff and once again there was a movement in the carriage as the passengers became aware of *Seacliff*, the station, and *Seacliff* the hospital, the asylum, glimpsed as a castle of dark stone between the hills. The train drew into the station. Yes, the loonies were there; everyone looked out at the loonies, known in Oamaru as those who were sent 'down the line', and in Dunedin, 'up the line'. Often it was hard to tell who were the loonies [p. 150].

> The six weeks I spent at Seacliff hospital in a world I'd never known among people whose existences I never thought possible, became for me a concentrated course in the horrors of insanity and the dwelling-place of those judged insane, separating me forever from the former acceptable realities and assurances of everyday life [p. 193].

> There was a personal geographical, even linguistic exclusiveness in this community of the insane, who yet had no legal or personal external identity – no clothes of their own to wear, no handbags, purses, no possessions but

a temporary bed to sleep in with a locker beside it, and a room to sit in and stare, called the *dayroom* [p. 193].

When I'd been home for a week or two my family grew less apprehensive in my presence – the change showed in the loosening of fear in their eyes; who knew what I might do; I was a loony, wasn't I? [p. 194].

I was again living the submissive, passive role which in hospital had been forced upon me but which my shy nature had accommodated with ease: at its best it is the role of the queen bee surrounded by her attendants; at its worst it is that of the victim without power or possession; and in both cases there is no ownership of one's self [p. 282].

Seabrook (1935) understood the nature of this passivity, and the seductiveness of it:

No responsibilities, no obligations, no problems to meet or solve, no duties or decisions. We didn't even have to decide when to get up in the morning or when to go to bed. Somebody else looked after us. Somebody else looked after everything. Lots of us had been grown up and responsible, meeting worries, problems, obligations, for twenty, thirty years. So that, cured now, outside where I have to decide everything for myself, I remember the haven it was – almost wish sometimes I were back there, back in the arms of my nut-college mother [p. 68].

The difference that was established first by social deviance and then deepened by diagnostic labelling and residence in an asylum were moral and spiritual not physical. There were no visible stigmata that determined who was insane and demarcated them from others. Yet, insidiously a gap opened up between those were designated as mentally ill and others. This gap could and often did close:

I became convinced, and still am, that functional mental derangement, generally speaking, has no physiological, facial, or cranial stigma … We were all cases who had gone off our trolleys, as it were, or had broken an axle, or had a monkey-wrench thrown in our gears, or had lost control, or had gone haywire, not *been* born so. And I assure you were indistinguishable to the naked eye from our keepers and attendants or from any average crowd outside, except when one, or a group of us started to do our special stuff [p. 96].

What I liked least at first in this Hall was my fellow-patients. They were too normal. They were nearly well, or getting well. They lived, talked, and deported themselves more or less as I imagine they always had outside, so that the social atmosphere was radically different from that of the hall below [p. 129].

Understandings of emotional disorders

Tim Lott's *The Scent of Dried Roses* (1996) was written in the wake of his mother's death by suicide. Lott had himself just recovered from a depressive episode before the death. In his book, he attempts to give meaning to both his mother's suicide and his own depression. In this, he is similar to other writers. Where he differs significantly is in the terms under which he operates. Whereas in *Out of Me,* Fiona Shaw (1997) predictably locates the problems in the internal world and in problematic relationships with her father, and Lewis Wolpert, in *Malignant Sadness* (1999), approaches the subject as a scientist, and a biological scientist at that, Lott prefers a social explanation. What he has in common with most writers on this subject is his refusal to accept that depression is merely the result of biochemical anomaly. For Lott, his mother's suicide and his own depression can both be understood as reflecting the decay of English self-confidence, loss of identity and the degradation of society during the 1970s and 1980s, exemplified by the deterioration of Southall, in London. This is a version of Durkheim's ideas about the social origins of human behaviour. Lott both enunciates his thesis and understands the problems with it and gives his explanations:

> There was the force of heredity, knitting with childhood experience. There was adult drama, sparking with the larger inner history of the old, old transformed country within which Jean was a tiny connection [p. 22].

> For Jean and me, when we plotted our own self-murders, our lives were good, better than most. We had friends, health, enough money, plenty of love. So what drove us to madness? Was it hidden and interior, some sickness of the brain? No – it was larger external powers, the flooding force of a disintegrating England, of mobility, dislocation, crumbling identity, separation, unbelonging, advancing relentlessly, too slow or massive to resist [p. 24].

> There is no trace of any aberration, any trust or wrinkle in Jean's childhood that might have curdled her inside, that might have tended her towards buried rage or desperate self-hatred, to be carried through life like a loaded gun in the bottom drawer [p. 58].

> If I was looking for some intellectual justification for imagining that the collapse of both my mother and myself may have been partly rooted in a wider crisis in England, Durkheim was a touchstone [p. 74].

> I didn't want to believe in depression, because it let the weak, the fuck-ups, the lazy and stupid off the hook, because it turned people into what they increasingly wanted to be: victims. And we were the C2s. We were not victims, we were conquerors. We were the new society of choice, and will, and endless, guilt-free shopping [p. 195].

> It doesn't add up, it doesn't cut a swathe that is clear. For if my mother and I were simply ill, am I not wasting everyone's time? England, history, family, love, regret, identity, meaning. Does their poetry fall apart under the prose of science? Is it as absurd as looking for the meaning of a headache in history, the meaning of cancer in culture? [p. 196].

It is clear that for Lott, depression cannot be merely the result of a perturbation in brain chemistry. Biochemical explanations will not do, social and psychological understanding, meaningful and symbolic understanding are what is required. This drive for meaning is most evident in psychiatry but it is not unknown in physical medicine. Patients with cancer also ask 'why me?' and are wont to resort to moral explanations.

Fiona Shaw (1997) expresses the same disquiet but from a different perspective:

> There was no scepticism and no psychology. Lives, it seems, can be described as illnesses and organised in just the same way as organic disease would be [p. 156].

Whilst 'postnatal depression' often arrives as though a bolt from the blue, it rises out of the fabric of each of our lives. And it's more deeply inscribed in the fabric of social life in our culture than is ever remotely acknowledged [p. 160].

The psychiatrists were never interested in the words I chose. Words had only one side to them, as far as they were concerned; storymaking was all very well so long as it didn't go too far ... So they found out very little about me, and so did I [p. 175].

But I was dismayed by the explanation Styron comes up with for it all. For most of his book he insists that depression is all in the body. It's a disease, an illness, a disorder, a question of neurotransmitters and hormones, something you leave to the biochemist rather than a biographer or autobiographer [p. 188].

When I am unhappy I often seem to myself like a mourner without an object for my grief. Until I discover and understand that object, I will go on keening, in the privacy of my own person [pp. 206–207].

What do these understandings or readings mean for psychiatrists? Unlike physicians, psychiatrists cannot ignore the social and personal meanings of illness. We cannot be indifferent to the compulsion that patients have for a coherent narrative of causation that moves outside the mechanistic materialism of biochemistry. For most patients, the explanations for their emotional disorder reside within the social world. Psychiatry does not need to adopt or even endorse these particular narrative explanations. However, our professional narratives of causation must at least be open to dialogue and, as individual clinicians, we must understand the motifs that are readily used by our patients.

Conclusion

Autobiographical accounts of the experience of psychiatric illness provide an insight into the nature of psychiatric disorders in a way that is not possible from standard psychiatric texts. The hope is that these accounts will help to enrich the language and thought of psychiatrists. The subjective, the personal, the social and cultural contexts are hallowed ground in autobiography, whereas in psychiatric texts it is the objective and general that is stamped and reinforced. The foregoing is only a fragment of what autobiographical narratives contain.

References

Beers, C. W. (1907) *A Mind that Found Itself. An Autobiography*. American Foundation for Mental Hygiene.

Ferguson, S. (1973) *A Guard Within*. Chatto & Windus.

Frame, J. (1961) *Faces in the Water*. Reprinted 1980. Women's Press.

Frame, J. (1983–85) *An Autobiography: To the Is-Land, An Angel at My Table and The Envoy from Mirror City*. Reprinted 1990. Women's Press.

Freud, S. (1911) Psycho-analytic notes on an autobiographical account of a case of paranoia (dementia paranoides). Reprinted (1953–1974) in the *Standard Edition of the Complete Psychological Works of Sigmund Freud* (trans. & ed. J. Strachey), vol. XII. Hogarth Press.

James, W. (1902) *The Varieties of Religious Experience*. Reprinted 1999. The Modern Library.

Jamison, K. R. (1995) *An Unquiet Mind. A Memoir of Moods and Madness*. Knopf.

Lott, T. (1996) *The Scent of Dried Roses*. Penguin.

Mill, J. S. (1873) *Autobiography*. Reprinted (1989): ed. J. M. Robson. Penguin.

Perceval, J (1838) *A Narrative of the Experience of a Gentleman during a State of Mental Derangement to Explain the Causes and the Nature of Insanity, and to Expose the Injudicious Conduct Pursued towards Many Sufferers under that Calamity*. Reprinted (1962) as *Perceval's Narrative* (ed. G. Bateson). Hogarth Press.

Sass, L. A. (1994) *The Paradoxes of Delusion. Wittgenstein, Schreber and the Schizophrenic Mind*. Cornell University Press.

Schreber, D. P. (1903) *Memoirs of My Nervous Illness*. Reprinted (1955): trans. I. Macalpine & R. A. Hunter. Wm. Dawson & Sons.

Seabrook, W. B. (1935) *Asylum*. Harrap.

Shaw, F. (1997) *Out of Me*. Penguin.

Styron, W. (1990) *Darkness Visible. A Memoir of Madness*. Cape.

CHAPTER 4

Fictional narrative and psychiatry

Femi Oyebode

Charlotte Brontë's novel *Jane Eyre*, published in 1847, sets the scene for how madness is perceived in society. It is a very popular work and the plight of Rochester's wife Bertha Mason is iconic of madness. Her fiendish laughter and screaming characterise her difference from others. Rochester is so ashamed of her that he has her locked away from human intercourse and keeps her presence a secret, signalling that madness is best kept out of sight. Bertha Mason's potential violence and the danger that she poses to Jane Eyre and Rochester link madness to violence very explicitly. The incurability of madness and the cost of providing specialised care and attention leave little room for optimism. Finally, the madwoman does not speak for herself, in other words, she is not granted the gift of speech that is the natural attribute of human beings. All in all, Bertha Mason, the madwoman, compels no compassion in us.

In this chapter, I explore the role of fictional narrative in shaping our knowledge, understanding and feelings about madness. It is impossible to give an exhaustive review of published novels that deal with the subject of madness: those examined here are only a means of exemplifying particular issues.

The amplification of deviance

Physical difference

Fictional narrative achieves its aims by making its characters stand out. This technique of magnifying aspects of characters in a novel can involve the amplification of physical characteristics, or the exaggeration of mannerisms, behaviour, speech or experience. One of the reasons insanity is of interest to writers is that already existent in the image of insanity is the implicit difference from others. When this difference is amplified, the result can be grotesque or a parody of what insanity is actually like. Cervantes' Don Quixote (1605) is an example of amplification of the physical characteristics of a subject that is then associated with his ineptitude, unusual thinking and behaviour. Quixote's ungainly appearance, his comical bearing, the 'mouldy and rust-eaten' suit of armour, which had been his great-great-grandfather's, and his less than healthy horse help to compose an image of the fool whose behaviour is rendered more comical because of the picture we already have of him. It is noteworthy that, although Don Quixote's madness is explicitly referred to in the book, the character is more in the line of the 'holy fool' described by Erasmus (1509). This method of amplifying physical characteristics is also used in *Jane Eyre*. Bertha Mason is the face of madness and she is described as follows:

> Fearful and ghastly to me oh sir, I never saw a face like it! It was a discoloured face – it was a savage face. I wish I could forget the roll of red eyes and the fearful blackened inflation of the lineaments! ... [It] was purple: the lips were swelled and dark; the brow furrowed; the black eye-brows widely raised over the blood-shot eyes, shall I tell you what it reminded me? ... of the foul German spectre and the Vampyre ... what it was, whether beast or human being, one could not, at first sight, tell: it grovelled, seemingly on all fours; it snatched and growled like some strange wild animal [Brontë, 1996 reprint: p. 317].

The association of the idea of madness with savagery and the less than human is clear. Brontë animalises, demonises and debases her. She is described as or like a 'condor', 'dog', 'goblin', 'wolf', 'hyena', 'fiend', 'hag', 'demon' and 'witch'. Mr Rochester tries to justify his attempt to take another wife by insisting that he 'had the right to break contact and seek sympathy with something at least human'. This 'inhuman' theme extends from animalising and demonising Bertha to rejecting her living existence when she is described as being dead, 'the ghastliness of living death'. She is also referred to as 'a corpse'.

In Patrick McGrath's novel *Spider* (1990), the protagonist's difference is symbolised by what he wears:

> I am wearing all my shirts and on top of them a black polo-neck jersey, and on top of that the jacket of my shabby grey suit. Suit trousers, thick grey socks (2 pairs), and a large pair of thick-soled black leather shoes with 10 close-set lace shoes ... I also have strips of brown wrapping paper and thin cardboard taped to my legs and torso, which crackle when I move [p. 151].

The protagonist dressed in this way in an attempt to prevent people from smelling the gas that he believed was seeping from his person.

However, the expected difference can itself be explored in such a way that madness can be made to inhabit an individual who shows no obvious stigmata, or at least the question can be asked whether any such stigmata exist. For example, in Janet Frame's autobiographical novel *Faces in the Water* (1961) the protagonist asks, 'I wondered if I had any distinguishing marks of madness about me?' (Frame, 1980 reprint: p. 58). Also, in V. S. Naipaul's novel *A House for Mr Biswas* (1961), Mr Biswas is not wild or violent, he makes no speeches and does not pretend to be driving a motor-car or picking cocoa, the two actions popularly associated with insanity. In this depiction of madness, he only looks exasperated and fatigued.

The aim of the writer in this mode is not merely to mark out what is alien, in the true sense of stigmatising – that is, to render visible by stigmata – but also to distance the reader from the symbol of madness. This distancing is necessary sometimes to reduce compassion for the character and at other times to deflect sympathy towards other characters. The risk always is that in portraying madness in this vein a more permanent disfigurement of the image of madness is achieved.

Psychological difference

Physical difference is only one aspect of the expected difference. Psychological difference is another. Here it is bizarre and unusual thinking processes that are paramount. Patrick McGrath's two novels *Asylum* and *Spider* trade in this currency. In *Asylum* (1996) McGrath explores the nature and consequences of jealousy, and in *Spider* (1990) he examines among other things the way that psychotic experience interferes with how the world is perceived. *Asylum* is as much about the social organisation of the asylum as it is an examination of sexual jealousy. As McGrath has commented, the story is a variation on Tolstoy's *Anna Karenina*: a psychiatrist's spouse has an affair with a patient, a transgression of social mores within a total institution (McGrath, 2002). As a study of morbid jealousy it succeeds. McGrath draws attention to the fact that delusional jealousy is justified by the production of trivial everyday occurrences as evidence: 'a flushing toilet, a stain on the floor, the placement of a box of washing powder on a window-sill' (McGrath, 1996: p. 8). Furthermore, the narrative voice comments:

> driven by morbid processes to suppose that his wife was betraying him with another man, he had reasoned first, that they must have ways of signalling their arrangements, and second, that their activities must leave traces. He had then manufactured evidence of such signals and traces from incidents as banal as her opening a window as a motorbike was going past in the street below, and from phenomena as insignificant as a crease in a pillow or a stain on a skirt [pp. 40–41].

Although the narrative in *Asylum* is compelling, it is in *Spider* that McGrath achieves his best effect. He manages to describe the world through the eyes of the protagonist, Spider, and the reader is taken in by the account. Spider's conviction of the reality of his beliefs and psychotic experiences convinces the reader too. Authorial coherence authenticates the narrative and makes Spider's account believable. It is true that Spider's world is never entirely explicable but none the less it has the compelling force of reality. It is a study of the architecture of psychotic experience. The struts and girders on which illusions, hallucinations and delusions are built are exposed. It is also a study of the mundane everyday life of an individual with chronic psychosis living in the community.

Perhaps the most impressive description of psychopathology relates to the experience of nihilistic delusions:

I was contaminated by it, it shrivelled me, it killed something inside me, made me a ghost, a dead thing, in short it turned me bad [McGrath, 1990: p. 97].

...for I am almost empty now, the foul taste in my mouth attests to this, and of course the smell of gas, and I wonder ... what they will find when they cut me open (if I'm not dead)? An anatomical monstrosity, surely: my intestine is wrapped tightly around the lower part of my spine and ascends in a taut snug spiral, thickening grossly into the colon about half-way up, which twists around my upper spine like a boa constrictor, the rectum passing through my skull and the anus issuing from the top of my head where an opening has been created between the bones joining the top of my skull, which I constantly finger in wondering horror, a sort of mature excretory fontanelle.

...a single thin pipe takes water from my stomach ... and this pipe alone drops through the void and connects to the thing between my legs that hardly resembles a formed male organ at all anymore [pp. 175–176].

What is remarkable is the accuracy of the psychopathology, and the question is whether McGrath could have achieved an insider's feel for madness without close study, as a child growing up in Broadmoor (where his father was the medical superintendent), of those around him – in other words, whether creative imagination alone can make the psychoses comprehensible. It is likely that personal experience of psychopathology or close contact with individuals who have it make for a more true-to-life characterisation of mental illness.

Gogol's *Diary of a Madman*, first published in 1834, describes the gradual mental disintegration of the narrator. The psychological deviance described is even more remarkable because we witness, as it were, the onset and steady progression of the decline. The diarist announces his experiences of hallucinations and his uncertainty about his identity:

quite recently I've started hearing and seeing things I'd never heard or seen before [1972 reprint: pp. 19–20].

I can't stand the smell of cabbage; the shops along Meshchanskaya just reek of it. What with this, and the infernal stench coming from under the front doors of all the houses, I held my nose and ran for all I was worth [p 25].

Why am I just a titular councillor? Perhaps I'm really a count or general and I'm merely imagining I'm a titular councillor? Perhaps I don't really know who I am at all? History has lots of examples of that sort of thing: there was some fairly ordinary man, not what you'd call a nobleman, but simply a tradesman or even a serf, and suddenly he discovered he was a great lord or a baron? [p 32].

Soon he becomes convinced that he is the King of Spain:

Today is a day of great triumph. There *is* a King of Spain. He has been found at last. That king is me. I only discovered this today. Frankly it all came to me in a flash. I cannot understand how I could even think or imagine for one moment I was only a titular councillor [pp. 33–34].

There are examples of neologisms: '86th Martober' (p. 34), 'Madrid, 30th Februarius' (p. 37). Also as the mental disintegration proceeds, the dates become more and more bizarre: 'April 43rd 2000' (p. 33), '86th Martober, between day and night' (p. 34), 'January in the same year falling after February' (p. 39), and 'De 34 te Mth eary' (p. 40). Once the primary delusion is established, the development of secondary delusions begins. For example, the diarist's explanation of his detention and transportation to an asylum is as follows:

> [S]o I'm in Spain now, and it was all so quick I hardly knew what was happening. This morning the Spanish deputation arrived and I got into a carriage with them ... We went at such a cracking pace we were at the Spanish frontier within half an hour [p. 37] ... a strange country Spain: in the first room I entered there were a lot of people with shaven heads [pp. 37–38].

Despite how he is treated, his primary delusion remains fixed and organises his subsequent beliefs:

> Up to this time Spain had been somewhat of a mystery to me. Their native customs and court etiquette are really most peculiar. I don't understand, I really do *not* understand them ... I think I'm safe in hazarding a guess that I've fallen into the hands of the Inquisition, and the person I thought was a minister of state was really the Grand Inquisitor himself. But I still don't understand how *kings* can be subjected to the Inquisition [p. 39].

Novels are not written as scientific studies of psychopathology. The novelist's interest in psychopathology is because of the intrinsic fascination that we all have for how the mind works, in either health or illness. However, for a story to work it has to be coherent and plausible. Therefore, psychopathology has to be comprehensible within the total structure of the narrative. Thus, even in an account of a disintegrating mind, the account still has to cohere. This means that Jaspers' notion of 'un-understandability' as a criterion for psychosis is usually breached in literature. There are, of course, researchers such as Bentall (2003) who argue that psychotic experiences are understandable. On the face of it, fictional accounts seem to agree with him, but I suspect that this is because of the need for fictional narrative to be comprehensible and coherent. *Diary of a Madman* is a good example of such an account written in the first person, in the voice of the madman, in which the disintegrating mind is yet able to give an account that coheres despite the often bizarre beliefs and behaviour of the diarist.

Violence

Violence is linked to madness in the minds of the laity. Partly, this link is reinforced by literature. Often the theme of jealousy is the device that makes the violence comprehensible. In *The Kreutzer Sonata*, published in 1889, Tolstoy explores the nature of marriage in Russian society using his own marriage as a model. His wife, Sonya, was reportedly hurt that Tolstoy's attack on marriage was based on private details of their own relationship. In the novel, through his narrator, he describes the end of affection, how 'sometimes I'd watch the way she poured her tea, the way she swung her leg or brought her spoon to her mouth; I'd listen to the little slurping noises she made as she sucked the liquid in and I used to hate her for that as for the most heinous crime' (Tolstoy, 1983 reprint: p. 74).

Tolstoy also describes the development of the jealousy of the narrator when his wife took on a new piano teacher. The account of the misinterpretation of trivial events and the imaginary changes in his wife bring to life the emotional basis and illogical reasoning that are characteristic of jealousy. This is similar to McGrath's account in *Asylum*. For example,

> I saw that right from that first meeting her eyes began to shine in a peculiar way and that, probably as a result of my jealousy, there was immediately established between them a kind of electric current which seemed to give their faces the same expression, the same gaze, the smile. Whenever she blushed or smiled, so did he [1996: p. 86].

> From the first moment that his eyes met those of my wife, I saw that the beast which lurked in them both, regardless of all social conventions and niceties, asked 'May I?', and replied 'Oh yes, certainly.' [p. 88].

> For the first time I felt a desire to give my animosity physical expression. I leapt to my feet and went up to her; I remember that at the very moment I got up I became aware of my animosity and asked myself whether it was a good thing for me to abandon myself to this feeling, and then told myself that it was a good thing, that it would give her a fright; ... 'Go or I'll kill you!' I shouted suddenly, going up to her and seizing her by the arm, consciously exaggerating the level of animosity in my voice. I must have appeared terrifying [p. 93].

> What was really so horrible was that I felt I had a complete and inalienable right to her body, as if it were my own, yet at the same time I felt that I wasn't the master of this body, that it did not belong to me, that she could do with it whatever she pleased, and that what she wanted to do with it wasn't what I wanted [p. 105].

So, it is clear that sexual jealousy is at least linked to the belief in proprietary rights over the spouse's body. In the end the narrator kills his wife:

> When people tell you they don't remember what they did when they are in a mad fit of rage, don't believe a word of it – it's all lies, nonsense. I remembered everything afterwards, and I've never ceased to remember it for one second. The more steam my rage got up, the more brilliantly the light of consciousness flared within me, making it impossible for me not to be aware of everything I was doing. I can't claim that I knew in advance what I was going to do, I was aware of each action I took at the moment I performed it, and sometimes, I think, a little before [p. 113].

> [I]t was only when I saw her dead face that I realised what I'd done. I realised that I'd killed her, that it was all my doing that from a warm, moving, living creature she'd been transformed into a cold, immobile waxen one, and that there was no setting to rights, not ever, not anywhere, not by any means [p. 118].

This association between madness and violence can, of course, refer to violence against the self. But it is the dramatic quality of violence against others that is most compelling and that is most often found in literature.

In Elfriede Jelinek's (1983) *The Piano Teacher*, the protagonist self-harms. Jelinek's writing style in this passage is an objective, observing authorial voice. Her syntax is deliberately awkward and she utilises unusual insertions of upper case within her sentences:

> When SHE's home alone, she cuts herself, slicing off her nose to spite other people's faces. She always waits and waits for the moment when she can cut herself unobserved. No sooner does the sound of the closing door die down than she takes out her little talisman, the paternal all-purpose razor. SHE peels the blade out of its Sunday coat of five layers of virginal plastic. She is very skilled in the use of blades; after all, she has to shave her father, shave that soft paternal cheek under the completely empty paternal brow, which is now undimmed by any thought, unwrinkled by any will. This blade is destined for HER flesh. This thin, elegant foil of bluish steel, pliable, elastic. SHE sits down in front of the magnifying side of the shaving mirror; spreading her legs, she makes a cut, magnifying the aperture that is the doorway into her body. She knows from experience that such a razor cut doesn't hurt, for her arms, hands, and legs have often served as guinea pigs. Her hobby is cutting her own body [1988 reprint: p. 86].

This account of self-inflicted harm directed at genitalia focuses on a rarely described aspect of self-harm. A hidden, secretive behaviour is given sufficient prominence that we cannot ignore it. There is no explanation for the self-inflicted harm to the body but it is set in the context of human life that is sad and impoverished of warmth. The protagonist dislikes herself, and although the self-harm is not explained as deriving from this the reader can deduce it from the story.

Again, as with the description of psychological deviance, the origin of violence must make sense, that is, must be understandable within the context of the narrative, even though the rationale need not be explicit. It is therefore unusual to have an account of motiveless violence. In Mario Vargas Llosa's novels *In Praise of the Stepmother* (1988) and *The Notebooks of Don Rigoberto* (1997), it is the damage, the violence to family life, that is evident. These novels about sexual preoccupation and fantasies are interesting enough from that viewpoint. But it is the ritualistic routines of Don Rigoberto, an obsessiveness not often met in novels, that is likely to be of most interest to psychiatrists:

> His ears were large and prominent; ... [although] as a child he was ashamed of their size and their downturned form, he had learnt to accept them. And now that he devoted one night a week to their care alone, he even felt proud of them ... He was removing the piliform excrescences from his right ear. All of a sudden he spied a stranger: the solitary little hair was swaying back and forth, disgustingly, in the centre of his neatly turned earlobe. He pulled it out with a slight jerk, and before throwing it into the washbasin to be flushed down the drain, he examined it with distaste [1998 reprint: pp. 23–26].

Out of sight

In *Jane Eyre*, Bertha Mason is locked away in the attic and supervised by Mrs Poole. The locking away in secrecy speaks partly to the shamefulness of having madness in the family. Unlike Bertha Mason, most people at that time (the mid-19th century) would have been detained in asylums. Writing in Vienna in the interwar years, Robert Musil describes an asylum in his 1931 novel *The Man without Qualities*:

> In this new ward a series of horrible apparitions crouched and sat in their beds, everything about their bodies crooked, unclean, twisted or paralysed. Decayed teeth. Waggling heads. Heads too big, too small, totally misshapen. Slack, drooping jaws from which saliva was dribbling, without food or words. Yard-wide leaden barriers seemed to lie between these souls and the world [1995 reprint: p. 1068].

He then likens an asylum to hell:

> Hell is not interesting, it is terrifying ... It is precisely the bare idea of an unimaginable and thereby inescapable everlasting punishment and agony, the premise of an inexorable change for the worse, impervious to any attempt to reverse it, that has the fascination of an abyss. Insane asylums are also like that. They are poorhouses. They have something of hell's lack of imagination [p. 1070].

The kind of asylum that Musil describes, a total institution with thousands of beds, is probably a thing of the past in most Western countries. However, the conditions within psychiatric hospitals and nursing homes may not have changed much since then.

The autobiographical novels *The Bell Jar* by Sylvia Plath (1963) and *Faces in the Water* by Janet Frame (1961) tackle the experience of institutional care. Plath, who herself suffered from depression and eventually killed herself, set her account in a private asylum in the USA, whereas Frame's account is set in two asylums in New Zealand. Both deal with how a patient experiences electroconvulsive treatment (ECT) in the period when unmodified ECT was routinely administered. Plath describes it as follows: 'then something bent down and took hold of me and shook me like the end of the world. Whee-ee-ee-ee-ee, it shrilled, through an air crackling with blue light, and with each flash a great jolt drubbed me till I thought my bones would break and the sap fly out of me like a split plant' (p. 151). Following the treatment, 'all the heat and fear had purged itself. I felt surprisingly at peace. The bell jar hung, suspended, a few feet above my head. I was open to the circulating air' (p. 227).

Frame's account likens ECT to death in the electric chair and suggests that far from being treatment it was a form of punishment, at least from the patient's point of view:

> [W]e know the rumours attached to EST [*sic*] – it is training for Sing Sing when we are at last convicted of murder and sentenced to death and sit strapped in the electric chair with the electrodes touching our skin through slits in our clothing; our hair is singed as we die and the last smell in our nostrils is the smell of ourselves burning. And the fear leads some patients to more madness [Frame, 1980 reprint: p. 23].

> Whether or not I was for shock treatment, the new and fashionable means of quieting people and making them realise that orders are to be obeyed and floors are to be polished without anyone protesting and faces are made to be fixed into smiles and weeping is a crime [p. 15].

49

Although these accounts of ECT are written for literary effect, the ideas and feelings that they transmit are important. As psychiatrists, it may be that we underestimate the fear and awe with which patients approach ECT. Familiarity with the treatment may be said to have bred in us not so much contempt as indifference, but given how feared ECT is as a treatment, the possibility of its misuse as a potent instrument of control and punishment is at least from the patient's point of view very real.

Both Plath and Frame describe the implications of having been in an asylum. For example, Plath says 'a lot of people would treat me gingerly, or even avoid me, like a leper with a warning bell' (Plath, 1963: p. 249) and one of her characters says 'I wonder whom you'll marry now, Esther. Now you've been in here' (p. 254). Frame's account documents the impact of institutionalisation: how the unkemptness of the old men 'showed from within, beyond the shabby appearance of their braces hitching their pants anyhow, their unbuttoned flies, their flannel shirts bunched out, hanging loose' (Frame, 1980 reprint: p. 50). How there were patients who had 'long ago given up attempts at speech and now made noises appropriate to their habitat: animal noises, whimpers; sometimes they bayed and howled like lonely dogs attending the moon' (p. 92). How easy it was to lose social graces because of the conditions of the wards and how, for example, the narrator would wet herself if she were refused permission to go to the lavatory. The particular hopelessness of the men is described as follows:

> I once looked through at the men prowling unshaven in their tattered outlaw clothes, and I could not forget their hopelessness; it seemed deeper than that of the women, for all the masculine power and pride were lost and some of the men were weeping and in our civilisation it seems that only a final terrible grief can reduce a man to tears (p. 170).

However, the despair and the forlorn air described in these accounts is balanced by McGrath's account of how dignity and communion are maintained:

> Even when a man has nothing to call his own he finds ways of acquiring possessions; he then finds ways of concealing his possessions from the attendants. What you did on a hard-bench ward was tie one end of a piece of string to a belt-loop, and the other end to the top of a sock, then have the sock dangle down inside of your trousers. In it you kept tobacco, sewing materials, pencil and paper, other bits of string – whatever you had that was of use or value [McGrath, 1996: p. 164].

> [N]o matter how deep a man may be sunk in his own melancholy, his own madness – adrift, you'd think, all lines to the social body cut – yet he'd never fail to give you his butt to light your own with, *there is no madness, so deep that it excludes you from the community of tobacco* [p. 140, my italics].

It may be that McGrath's different and more optimistic perspective, compared with Plath and Frame, is attributable to the fact he was never a patient in an asylum. Rather, he lived in one as a child and worked in another in adulthood, as a nursing assistant.

Asylum life was regulated by nurses and dictated by doctors. The relationship of patients to nurses and to doctors therefore forms a significant part of the accounts of the nature of the rhythm and life in asylums. The rare sighting of doctors on the wards and the precious little time that they had for patients are all well captured by Frame:

> the doctor would pause sometimes to inquire, smiling in a friendly manner, but at the same time glancing hastily at his watch and perhaps wondering how in the hour before lunch he could possibly finish his rounds of all the women's wards and get back to his office to deal with correspondence and interviews with demanding puzzled alarmed ashamed relatives [1980 reprint, p. 28].

As for nurses, because they were overworked they had become 'sadistic custodians' (p. 98) and were 'most of the time without compassion' (p. 106) and harassed and reluctant carers. Frame's account is set in New Zealand between the First and Second World Wars, yet the pressures on the wards have a contemporary feel. What one hopes is that the indifference, ruthlessness and sadism are things of the past.

Frame also describes how it feels not to be consulted about her treatment and likely fate. She writes: 'I felt remote from the arrangements being made for me; as if I were lying on my death bed watching the invasion of my house and the disposal of my treasures and glimpsing through the half-open door into the adjoining room the waiting coffin' (p. 216). Yet, the plans concern lobotomy and the thought of the operation becomes for her a nightmare: 'today they will seize me, shave my head, dope me, send me to the hospital in the city, and when I open my eyes ... the thieves wearing gloves and with permission and delicacy, have entered and politely ransacked the storehouse and departed calm and unembarrassed' (p. 216).

This account emphasises the tremendous authority and power that doctors have in relation to patients and their treatment. And how passive and uninvolved the patient may feel, and how inevitable they may see the treatment regimens. Patients in this environment were very aware of their status. They were aware of the requirement to conform to the asylum's norms and conventions because these determined whether life would be easy or not. They were also often lonely with little meaningful activity and very impoverished social life:

> Were we not the 'sensibly ill' who did not yet substitute animal noises for speech or fling our limbs in uncontrolled motion or dissolve into secret silent hilarity? [p. 19].

> When I first came to Cliffhaven and walked into the dayroom and saw the people sitting and staring, I thought, as a passerby in the street thinks when he sees someone staring into the sky, If I look up too, I will see it. And I looked but I did not see it. And the staring was not, as it is in the streets, an occasion for crowds who share the spectacle; it was an occasion of loneliness, of vision on a closed private circuit [p. 20].

> There is no past, present or future. Using tenses to divide time is like chalk marks on water. I do not know if my experiences at Cliffhaven happened years ago, are happening now, or lie in wait for me in what is called the future [p. 37].

And at times I murmured the token phrase to the doctor, 'When can I go home?' Knowing that home was a place where I least desired to be. They would watch me for signs of abnormality, like ferrets around a rabbit burrow waiting for the rabbit to appear [p. 38].

You learned with earnest expectation to 'fit in'; you learned not to cry in company but to smile and pronounce yourself pleased, and ask from time to time if you could go home, as proof that you were getting better and therefore in no need of being smuggled in the night to ward 2 [p. 40].

The gift of speech

Bertha Mason did not utter any intelligible speech in *Jane Eyre*. It took Jean Rhys's (1966) novel *Wide Sargasso Sea* to give her voice. Bertha Mason derived from a Creole Caribbean family, and Rhys's novel is set in the West Indies and drew on the author's understanding of the position of planter families following the Emancipation. In Rhys's novel, Bertha Mason emerges as a woman, a person, with motivation and life goals within the strictures of a woman's life in the West Indies and England of the 19th century. Rhys undercuts the impression created in *Jane Eyre* that madness is inextricably linked to a lack of logical and comprehensible motivation. The Bertha Mason in *Wide Sargasso Sea* compels our compassion and understanding. It is Rochester whose motivation and behaviour are less than honourable.

Both Edward Said (1993) and Chinua Achebe (1988) have drawn our attention to the fact that literature tells us as much by what is taken for granted or left out as it does by what is written. For example, in Conrad's *Heart of Darkness* (1899), the African viewpoint is unrepresented, so that, indirectly, the humanity of the African population is denied, simply by denying them a voice in the narrative. The same sort of thing seems to be the case in *Jane Eyre*. Although it could be argued that it is accidental that Bertha Mason is a Creole woman, this is unlikely to be the case. It is more likely that her being alien to England makes her alienation, her madness, more acceptable. It is as if Brontë were saying, 'Having resided in foreign and hot climes such as the Caribbean, it is no wonder that Bertha Mason is mad!' Feminist readings of *Jane Eyre* emphasise the fact that it is the patriarchal arrangements of 19th-century England that explain Bertha Mason's madness. So, for example, in 1979 Gilbert & Gubar argued that

> the problems encountered by the protagonist as she struggles from the imprisonment of her childhood toward an almost unthinkable goal of mature freedom are symptomatic of difficulties Everywoman in a patriarchal society must meet and overcome: oppression (at Gateshead), starvation (at Lowood), madness (at Thornfield), and coldness (at Marsh End) [Gilbert & Gubar, 1984 reprint: p. 339].

This line of reasoning usually supports its thesis by pointing to narratives such as C. P. Gilman's 1899 novel *The Yellow Wallpaper* to validate its case. Gilman explains that she wrote the book against the advice of her psychiatrist, the famous S. Weir Mitchell, that she 'live as domestic a life as far as possible'. In opposition to him, Gilman went to work on the novella, a narrative based on her own experience of mental illness, because work is 'the normal life of every human being' and without it 'one is a pauper and a parasite' (Gilman, 1998 reprint). In her novel Gilman describes the progression to puerperal psychosis. It is undeniable that the structures of patriarchal society deny women freedom and economic autonomy. How far these structures are responsible for psychosis is a moot point. But it is clear from fictional narratives based on autobiographical experience that there were people who had 'long ago given up attempts at speech and now made noises appropriate to their habitat' (Frame, 1980 reprint: p. 92). This loss of speech was compounded by the attitude of society to the insane:

> ... on leaving the hospital you were not immediately discharged but placed on probation, as if you committed a criminal offence, so that you might be away from the hospital and still be legally insane, unable to vote, to sign papers or travel abroad [1980 reprint: p. 43].

> I wondered if I had any distinguishing marks of madness about me, and I wondered if the people understood or wanted to understand what lay beyond the station [Cliffhaven], up the road over the cattle stop and up the winding path and behind the locked doors of the gray stone building [p. 58].

> They were not sure how to talk to us or what to say, they had learned somewhere that a fixed smile was necessary, therefore they smiled ... They did not seem to be able to make up their minds whether we were deaf or dumb or mentally defective, so when they spoke they raised their voices and moved their lips with exaggerated care and their vocabulary was the simplest, in case we did not understand [p. 162].

Frame describes the delight of returning to world of everyday speech: 'It was strange to be amongst people who talked, and at first I could not grasp the idea of talking, making sentences aloud, entering conversation, shunting back and forth with words in the once-darkened carriages lit with meaning' (p. 221).

Conclusion

Beveridge (2003) has rehearsed a number of arguments in favour of reading literature. He highlights how literature allows psychiatrists to engage imaginatively with the lives and inner worlds of a larger number of individuals, albeit that they are fictional; how a bioscientific model offers a limited and indeed an impoverished description of human life; and how literature may at least aid our empathic and ethical capacity. He also draws attention to the fact that literature is not written with clinical application in mind. What is obvious is that madness and abnormal human experience and behaviour are of great interest to writers. Whether psychiatrists read them or not, these fictional accounts will undoubtedly influence how wider society perceives mental illness, how they react to it and, ultimately, how governments respond by way of policy. Novels are revealing insofar as what is implicit in them, the unexplained and unexamined context, tells us something about the assumptions that cultures make about mental illness. But novels may also ignore aspects of madness because 'it would damage the romantic popular idea of the insane as a person whose speech appeals as immediately poetic' (Beveridge, 2003). Fictional literature is an attempt to create and reflect, using the imagination, the world we as psychiatrists know well. It gives us the opportunity to stand back from that world, to contemplate it, before once again immersing ourselves in it, for better or worse. And unlike the advice given to Janet Frame by one her nurses, 'When you leave hospital you must forget all you have ever seen, put it out of your mind completely as if it never happened, and go and live a normal life in the outside world' (Frame, 1981: p. 254), we want to value the world we know well and use fictional accounts to better understand it.

References

Achebe, C. (1988) *Hopes and Impediments*. Heinemann.

Bentall, R. P. (2003) *Madness Explained*. Allen Lane.

Beveridge, A. (2003) Should psychiatrists read fiction? *British Journal of Psychiatry*, **182**, 385–387.

Brontë, C. (1847) *Jane Eyre*. Reprinted 1996. Penguin.

Cervantes, M. (1605) *Don Quixote*. Reprinted (1999): trans. C. Jarvis. Oxford University Press.

Erasmus, D. (1509) *Stultitiae Laus*. Reprinted (1971) as *In Praise of Folly* (trans. B. Radice). Penguin Books.

Frame, J. (1961) *Faces in the Water*. Reprinted 1980. Women's Press.

Gilbert, S. M. & Gubar, S. (1979) *The Madwoman in the Attic. The Woman Writer and Nineteenth Century Literary Imagination*. Reprinted 1984. Yale University Press.

Gilman, C. P. (1899) *The Yellow Wallpaper*. Reprinted (1998): ed. D. M. Bauer. Bedford Books.

Gogol, N. (1834) *Zapiski sumashedshego*. Reprinted (1972) as *Diary of a Madman and Other Stories* (trans. R. Wilks). Penguin Books.

Jelinek, E. (1983) *Die Klavierspielerin*. Reprinted (1988) as *The Piano Teacher* (trans. J. Neugroschel). Serpent's Tail.

McGrath, P. (1990) *Spider*. Penguin.

McGrath, P. (1996) *Asylum*. Viking.

McGrath, P. (2002) Problem of drawing from psychiatry for a fiction writer. *Psychiatric Bulletin*, **26**, 140–143.

Musil, R. (1931) *Der Mann ohne Eigenschaften*. Reprinted (1995) as *The Man without Qualities* (trans. S. Wilkins). Picador.

Plath, S. (1963) *The Bell Jar*. Faber & Faber.

Rhys, J. (1966) *Wide Sargasso Sea*. Penguin Books.

Said, E. (1993) *Culture and Imperialism*. New York: Vintage Books.

Tolstoy, L. (1889) *Kreutzerova sonata*. Reprinted (1983) as *The Kreutzer Sonata* (trans. D. McDuff). Penguin Books.

Vargos Llosa, M. (1997) *Los cuadernos de don Rigoberto*. Reprinted (1998) as *The Notebooks of Don Rigoberto* (trans. E. Grossman). Faber & Faber.

CHAPTER 5

Poetry and psychiatry

Femi Oyebode

Poetry is not easy to define. It is not merely verse, which is only the formal convention or structure in which poetry is expressed. So, we can have verse written in particular metric forms, yet still be missing whatever the essential quality is that we describe as poetry. It was once not uncommon for lectures or scientific reports to be written in verse and no one would have mistaken the product for poetry. So, what is poetry? Valéry goes some way in attempting to capture the essence of poetry. He argues that poetry is affiliated to song, that it is integral to the language used in its expression, and that it relies on the human voice and ear. And that it is also the means by which emotions and passion are expressed:

> The interest in prose writings is, as it were, apart from the writing themselves and born of the consumption of the text, – the interest in poems is an integral part of the poems and can never be separated from them [Valéry, 1950: p. 148].

> In song the words tend to lose their significance, do often lose it, while at the extreme, in current prose it is the musical value that tends to disappear – so that verse stands symmetrically, as it were, between song, on the one hand, and prose on the other – and is thus admirably and delicately balanced between the sensual and the intellectual power of language [p. 157].

> For a long, long time the human voice was the foundation and condition of literature. The presence of the voice explains the earliest literature from which classical literature derived its form and its admirable temperament. The whole human body present beneath the voice, as a support and necessary balance for the idea … Then came the day when people knew how to read with their eyes, without spelling out the words, without hearing, and literature was thereby entirely altered [p. 149].

> [Poetry] is the attempt to represent, or to restore, by means of articulated language those things, or that thing, which cries, tears, caresses, kisses, sighs, etc., try obscurely to express, and which objects seem to want to express in all that is lifelike in them or appears to have design [p. 147].

This latter point, the aspect of poetry that is to do with the expression of passion and emotions, draws out why poetry can be so important in the psychiatric context. Love and loss both seem to be much the ready source of inspiration for poetry. Love and loss are also quite central to many of the

55

circumstances that psychiatrists face. The close connection between poetry and language is emphasised by T. S. Eliot (1957) as follows: 'We may say that the duty of the poet, as poet, is only indirectly to his people: his direct duty is to his language, first to preserve, and second to extend and improve' (p. 20). It is worth emphasising therefore that for poets language matters, whereas for other writers language is merely the tool, the instrument with which ideas and stories are expressed.

In this chapter, the aim is to examine and explore the poems of poets who have had experience of psychiatric disorders. I intend to see how the poems describe the manifold experiences of emotional anguish, the nature of psychiatric institutions and relationships with doctors and others. Poetry is often able to speak directly and cogently, to get to the heart of a subject in a few choice words, to draw us into the spirit of the moment, to engage our attention and empathy, and ultimately render visible the humanity in particular experiences. Here I mean by humanity, the vulnerability of the subjects of experience and our solidarity with them as fellow human beings.

Waiting rooms and wards

There is a sense in which poems are to novels as photographs are to motion films; this is the facility of the poem to focus on the incidental or small and to magnify it or to slow down it in order to render what has become commonplace and banal, fresh and once more memorable. Very much as a still photograph does. This aspect of poetry is clearly in evidence in the poems of Elizabeth Jennings (1926–2001), particularly in the poems that deal with her experience of hospitalisation. She is known to have had an episode of illness in 1961. In the poem 'A mental hospital sitting-room' (Jennings, 2002 reprint: pp. 72–73) she wrote:

> Utrillo on the wall. A nun is climbing
> Steps in Montmartre. We patients sit below.

These introductory two lines to the poem fix our attention to the ubiquitous habit of decorating the walls of psychiatric hospitals with reproductions of paintings. The poem continues,

> It is as if a scream were opened wide,
> A mouth demanding everyone to listen.
> Too many people cry, too many hide
> And stare into themselves. I am afraid.
> There are no life-belts here on which to fasten.

The desolation of the sitting-room is palpable. There is also the sheer fact that the anguish of each person competes for and demands attention but solace is not forthcoming. She concludes,

> The only hope is visitors will come
> And talk of other things than our disease …
> So much is stagnant and yet nothing dies.

In 'VI Hospital', from the series of poems entitled 'Sequence in hospital' (2002 reprint: p. 65), she wrote:

> Observe the hours which seem to stand
> Between these beds and pause until
> A shriek breaks through the time to show
> That humankind is suffering still.

Jennings has the gift to make salient that which we may have become inured to. Very quickly after coming to work in psychiatry, the screams and shrieks, these visible symptoms of human sorrow, can become part of the background noise that one becomes indifferent to. It is also the case that the intensity of the long unproductive hours, the burden of these hours that patients endure, is not properly appreciated. Jennings in her simple lines 'Observe the hours which seem to stand/Between these beds…' somehow works the magic of restoring to us our fresh and sensitive selves so that we can see the world as it is for the patient who endures these hours.

The poem continues,

> A world where silence has no hold
> Except a tentative small grip.
> Limp hands upon the blankets fold,
> Minds from their bodies slowly slip.
>
> Though death is never talked of here.
> It is more palpable and felt –
> Touching the cheek or in a tear –
> By being present by default.
>
> The muffled cries, the curtains drawn,
> The flowers pale before they fall –
> The world itself is here brought down
> To what is suffering and small.

In another poem from the series 'Sequence in hospital' (2002 reprint: p. 64) Jennings wrote,

> Like children now, bed close to bed,
> With flowers set up where toys would be
> In real childhoods, secretly
> We cherish each our own disease,
> And when we talk we talk to please
> Ourselves that still we are not dead.

Here we are drawn to the 'flowers' and from that to the 'secret', the cherishing of personal infirmity as once soldiers were wont to be proud of their war wounds.

These poems by Elizabeth Jennings are remarkable not least because they are written following her recovery but also because they demonstrate, if nothing else can, that the comprehending and observing intelligence remains alert during periods of serious illness. The intelligence continues to register and organise experiences. This is a salutary lesson for all clinicians. In the poem 'Night sister' (2002 reprint: p. 74), Jennings writes of her admiration of and gratitude to a ward sister. But more significantly, she shows that patients care for and have concerns for the welfare of those that look after them:

> How is it possible not to grow hard,
> To build a shell around yourself when you
> Have to watch so much pain, and hear it too?
> Many you see are puzzled, wounded; few
> Are cheerful long. How can you not be scarred?

> To view a birth or death seems natural,
> But these locked doors, these sudden shouts and tears
> Graze all the peaceful skies. A world of fears
> Like the ghost-haunting of the owl appears.
> And yet you love that stillness and that call.

Administering madness

Poetry is able to create an atmosphere, that is, to build a word picture that includes not simply the description of a place but creates the texture, colour, smell and pace of a situation. How exactly poetry achieves these effects is unclear but it certainly involves the use of the musical aspects of language: rhyme, assonance, rhythm, pace and the physicality of the word. This is the way the word both sounds to the ear and feels sensually to say, to mouth. In addition to these properties of language, words are able to carry baggage across generations and across peculiarities of use. These resonances add to how language can come to create a particular sense, a texture of emotion that does not appear to be obvious in a superficial reading of a line.

Eliot (1957) in his essay 'The music of poetry' remarks that 'the whole poem need not be, and often should not be wholly melodious' (p. 32). He develops his argument by indicating that 'The ugly words are the words not fitted for the company in which they find themselves' (p. 32). Here Eliot is making the point that accuracy of word choice, diction, is as much about the other words that a word is required to keep company with. Robert Lowell (1917–1977), an American poet from an illustrious Boston family, is regarded as perhaps the most European (or some would say English) of his American contemporaries. Lowell is known to have had bipolar mood disorder and was hospitalised on several occasions. Technically adept, formally rigorous and with an extensive diction, Lowell's poetry is classified as 'confessional'. He influenced Sylvia Plath and Anne Sexton. In his last volume of poetry *Day by Day* (Lowell, 1975) he wrote of his experience of detention under the Mental Health Act in London in the poem 'Visitors' (pp. 110–111):

> To no good
> they enter at right angles and on the run –
> two black verticals are suddenly four
> ambulance drivers in blue serge,

or the police doing double-duty.
They comb our intimate, messy bedroom,
scrutinize worksheets
illegible with second-thoughts,
then shed them in their stride,
as if they owned the room. They do.
They crowd me and scatter – inspecting
my cast-off clothes for clues?
They are fat beyond the call of duty –
with jocose civility,
they laugh at everything I say:

In these lines Lowell helps us to see that the ambulance drivers and
policemen intrude into his privacy. This is not an anti-psychiatry tract but a
well-observed piece of writing that succeeds in both inviting us and showing
how intrusive our response to this invitation is, for we are like the policemen albeit invited in. We feel embarrassment and shame at the intrusion.
Lowell's language, in this poem, is not melodious. It is angular and jerky
but it suits the temper of the poem. Lowell concludes,

I follow my own removal,
stiffly, gratefully even, but without feeling.
Why has my talkative
teasing tongue stopped talking?
My detachment must be paid for,
tomorrow will be worse than today,
heaven and hell will be the same –
to wait in foreboding
without the nourishment of drama...
assuming, then as now,
this didn't happen to me –
my little strip of eternity.

Lowell like Jennings is also interested in his fellow patients. He remarks
in the poem 'Home', 'the trouble is the patients are tediously themselves'
(p. 113) and then goes on to describe two patients:

The painter who burned both hands
after trying to kill her baby, says,
'Is there no one in Northampton
who goes to the Continent in the winter?'
The alcoholic convert keeps smiling,
'Thank you, Professor, for saving my life;
you taught me homosexuality is a heinous crime.'
I hadn't. I'm a thorazined fixture
in the immovable square-cushioned chairs
for seconds like migrant birds.

Lowell starts the final stanza,

The immovable chairs have swallowed up the patients,
and speak with the eloquence of emptiness.
By each the same morning paper lies unread [...]

These observations of the people and environment recall Jennings' description of the sitting-room and wards. And refracted in these observations are the patients' responses to their environment, something that is rarely inquired into in clinical psychiatry. The physical environment is usually taken for granted and the relationship between patients on a fast-paced ward is not even glossed over: it is just ignored.

The ritual of the asylum dance features in fiction (see Patrick McGrath's 1996 *Asylum*) and in autobiography (see William Seabrook's 1935 *Asylum*). John Burnside's poem 'The asylum dance' (Burnside, 2006a: pp. 56–57) provides the opportunity for a narrative poem to explore how the inmates of an asylum are seen by visitors; this is in contrast to the approach of Jennings and Lowell, discussed above, who write directly out of experience and do not attempt to conceal this fact. Burnside too has been in psychiatric hospitals, but not, I believe, in the period of asylum dances. His poetical approach to the subject allows a measure of distance from his own personal experience, his periods in asylums, that he has already written about in *A Lie about My Father* (Burnside, 2006b).

The poem begins:

> At one time, I looked forward to the dance:
> wandering back and forth in the quiet
> heat of an August morning,
> packing the car with cup cakes and lemonade,
> boxes of plums or cherries, petits-fours,
> nuts and spice cake, mousse and vol-au-vents.

The scene is at once set for the annual pilgrimage to the local asylum:

> It was something we did, every year,
> in that backwater town, abandoning our lawns and flower beds,
> to meet the patients, out at Summerswood.

And the poem continues,

> It seemed a privilege to be allowed
> within those gates, and know we might return,
> to see the meadows, striped with light and shade,
> the silent lake, the fallen cedar trees.
> We went there for the dance: a ritual
> of touch and distance, webs of courtesy
> and guesswork; shifts
> from sunlight into shade;
> and when the patients came downstairs
> to join us, smiling, utterly polite,
> in new-pressed clothes, like cousins twice-removed,
> they had the look of people glimpsed in mirrors,
> subtle as ghosts, yet real, with the vague
> good-humour of the lost.
> How we appeared to them, I can only imagine:
> too solid, perhaps, too easy with ourselves,
> sure of our movements, blessed with a measured desire.

Burnside evokes a wistful and charming setting, even an enchanting, picturesque occasion. The risk is that madness and the asylum can come to be romanticised. It is true that the asylum, set as it was in the country, with a grand exterior and perfectly cut lawns, can seem to the eye an idyll, a place that refreshes and restores. But this is only part of the story. In comparing the visitors to the patients Burnside is already clarifying the boundaries, delineating difference and suggesting that the asylum is a foreign and alien country. He writes about 'townsfolk conferring the weight of a normal world', and goes on 'Beside the patients, we were lithe and calm'. This is to say that the townsfolk were distinguishable from the patients, that madness has a mark, that it stigmatises and that the stigma influences movement and dance, rendering graceless those afflicted. Burnside, no doubt, has no intention to stigmatise. He is simply narrating a story that needs a particular colour and texture. He continues:

> We loved them for the way they witnessed us
> standing in twos and threes in the waning light,
> made other by the rhythm of the dance,
> the pull of a larger world, and that taste on the air
> of birchwood and streams; that knowledge of ourselves
> as bodies clothed in brightness, moving apart
> and coming together, cooling
> slowly, as the lawn and rose-beds cooled.

Melancholia and despair

Poetry is particularly well suited to the expression of intense emotions such as sadness and love. This is why poetry is both written and read in response to grief or new-found love. It speaks directly and somehow articulates the depth of feeling. It can give words to inchoate feeling, helping to structure feeling so that it can be better handled by language. Or, simply, it can allow recognition that the feelings are not unique but understood and experienced by others. This can reduce the sense of isolation that passion or despair can create. The risk for the poet is that the emotion may overwhelm and distort the structure rather than be constrained and put at the service of the poem. All art is aimed at structuring and communicating emotion and dictating the terms of the expression.

Ivor Gurney was born in Gloucester in 1890. He began composing music at an early age and won a scholarship to study music at the Royal College of Music in London in 1911. He was a contemporary of Vaughan Williams. He served in the First World War and was wounded and gassed. He is known to have suffered bipolar mood disorder from early adulthood, even before serving in the war. He was declared insane in 1922 and spent the rest of his life in the City of London asylum, where he died in 1937 from tuberculosis. In several poems Gurney describes his feelings of despair, of melancholia, of a wish for death. In 'To God' (Gurney, 1982 reprint: p. 197) he wrote:

61

Why have you made life so intolerable
And set me between four walls, where I am able
Not to escape meals without prayer, for that is possible
Only by annoying an attendant. And tonight a sensual
Hell has been put on me, so that all has deserted me
And I am merely crying and trembling in heart
For Death, and cannot get it. And gone out is part
of sanity. And there is dreadful hell within me.
And nothing helps. Forced meals there have been and electricity
And weakening of sanity by influence
That's dreadful to endure. And there is Orders
And I am praying for death, death, death,
And dreadful is the indrawing or out-breathing of breath,
Because of the intolerable insults put on my whole soul,
Of the soul loathed, loathed, loathed of the soul.
Gone out every bright thing from my mind.
All lost that ever God himself designed.
Not half can be written of cruelty of man, on man.
Not often such evil guessed as between Man and Man.

In another poem, 'The Shame' (1982 reprint: p. 205), Gurney says:

but this is dreadfulness beyond name.

Each minute packed with a badness beyond words,
The brain, the mind tortured as blind stones would do.

And, in 'An Appeal for Death' (p. 271), he wrote:

There is one who all day wishes to die,
And appeals for it – without a reason why –
Since Death is easy if men are merciful.
Water and land with chances are packed full.

These lines by Gurney draw us directly into what the experience of despair is like. Even for a poet of Gurney's skill, the actual experience appears to defy description and the usual appeal to metaphor or analogy fails in this context, but yet the anguish is true and real enough.

There are other approaches to the problem of describing what despair and despondency are like. Stevie Smith was born in Hull in 1902. We know that the family was abandoned by her father when she was 3 years old and that when she was 5 years old she developed tuberculosis and spent a protracted period at a sanatorium. She is reported as saying that her preoccupation with death started at 7 years of age. She is known to have cut her wrists and spent time in hospital in 1953. It was as if Smith was compelled to write about death and always beneath her humour and lightness of approach was this undertow. In 'Not waving but drowning' (Smith, 1975 reprint: p. 167) she wrote:

Nobody heard him, the dead man,
But still he lay moaning:
I was much further out than you thought
And not waving but drowning.

Poor chap, he always loved larking
And now he's dead
It must have been too cold for him his heart gave way,
They said.

Oh, no no no, it was too cold always
(Still the dead one lay moaning)
I was much too far out all my life
And not waving but drowning.

There is regret here in this poem and the obvious feeling of being alienated from what is going on for others in life. This sense of regret at having died, of failing to correctly call on the attention of others, of the message and the desire for rescue having been misread strikes at the heart. This is a picture of a misunderstood person and the misunderstanding results in death.

In 'The hostage' (pp. 185 and 186), we hear Smith say:

Even as a child, said the lady, I recall in my pram
Wishing it was over and done with. Oh I am
Already at fault. Wonderful how 'bright' they keep,
I'd say of other children, quite without rancour, then turn again to sleep.

And

Of course I never formed any close acquaintance.
Marriage? Out of the question. Well for instance
It might be infectious, this malaise of mine (an excuse?). Spread
That? I'd rather be dead.

In 'Come, Death (1)' (p. 70) she wrote

Why dost thou dally, Death, and tarry on the way?
When I have summoned thee with prayer and tears, why dost thou stay?
Come, Death, and carry now my soul away.

Wilt thou not come for calling, must I show
Force to constrain thy quick attention to my woe?
I have a hand upon thy Coat, and will
Not let thee go.

In these poems, we glimpse the preoccupying force of despair and how it spreads its shadow like a pall over everything else in the person's life. This compelling aspect of the wish for death is also present in the writing of Anne Sexton.

Anne Sexton (1928–1974) was born in Newton, Massachusetts. She experienced recurrent depressive illness and had a number of psychiatric hospital admissions. She died by her own hand in 1974. Sexton is regarded a confessional poet and was influenced by Lowell. In 'Wanting to die' (Sexton, 1988 reprint: pp. 98–99) she wrote:

Since you ask, most days I cannot remember.
I walk in my clothing, unmarked by that voyage.
Then the almost unnameable lust returns.

Even then I have nothing against life.
I know well the grass blades you mention,
the furniture you have placed under the sun.

> But suicides have a special language.
> Like carpenters they want to know *which tools*.
> They never ask *why build*.

She concludes:

> :
>
> Death's a sad bone; bruised, you'd say,
>
> and yet she waits for me, year after year,
> to so delicately undo an old wound,
> to empty my breath from its bad prison.

This 'lust' or passionate desire for death is akin to sexual desire, with the promise of resolution and satisfaction, and it can have the same grip on the imagination as sexual desire. In 'The addict' (Sexton, 1988 reprint: pp. 114–115), Sexton also makes the connection with compulsive urgency, the craving for an addictive substance:

> Don't they know that I promised to die!
> I'm keeping in practice.
> I'm merely staying in shape.
> The pills are a mother, but better,
> every color and as good as sour balls.
> I'm on a diet from death.
>
> :
>
> Yes
> I try
> to kill myself in small amounts,
> an innocuous occupation.
> Actually I'm hung up on it.
> But remember I don't make too much noise.
> And frankly no one has to lug me out
> and I don't stand there in my winding sheet.

Playfulness or prayer

Tone is important in poetry. This is probably best exemplified by the role of tone in music. For example, John Coltrane's commitment can be characterised by the earnestness in his playing of each note, as if his life depended on it. The same can be said of the pure, virginal tone of Ella Fitzgerald's singing, the elegance and suaveness of Miles Davis, or Billie Holliday's intense sorrowful tone. In poetry, tone, when it characterises the totality of a poet's writing, can be identified as the poet's voice. Some poets have a characteristic playfulness or earnestness: Stevie Smith, for example, wrote with a particular playfulness masking an intrinsic seriousness and anguish. Sexton, too, often wrote in this key. In 'Clothes' (1988 reprint: pp. 216–217) she wrote:

> Put on a clean shirt
> before you die, some Russian said.

Nothing with drool, please,
no egg spots, no blood,
no sweat, no sperm.
You want me clean, God,
so I'll try to comply.

This is a light-hearted poem about dressing in preparation for suicide and it belies the morbidity of the subject. She concludes:

For underpants I'll pick white cotton,
the briefs of my childhood,
for it was my mother's dictum
that nice girls wore only white cotton.
If my mother had lived to see it
she would have put a WANTED sign up in the post office
for the black, the red, the blue I've worn.
Still, it would be perfectly fine with me
to die like a nice girl
smelling of Clorox and Duz.
Being sixteen-in-the-pants
I would die full of questions.

In contrast to the playful tone that Sexton adopts, other poets have an earnestness that is expressed in prayer form. It is as if melancholia and despair call forth spiritual crisis, to which the only appropriate and adequate response is that of prayer.

John Berryman (1914–1972) died by suicide. His poem 'Eleven addresses to the Lord' (Berryman, 1989 reprint: p. 215) reveals this inclination:

Master of beauty, craftsman of the snowflake,
inimitable contriver,
endower of Earth so gorgeous & different from the boring Moon,
thank you for such as it is my gift.

I have made up a morning prayer for you
containing with precision everything that most matters.
'According to Thy will' the thing begins.
It took me off & on two days. It does not aim at eloquence.

You have come to my rescue again & again
in my impassable, sometimes despairing years.
You have allowed my brilliant friends to destroy themselves
and I am still here, severely damaged, but functioning.

The same sentiment appears to underlie Jennings' poem 'Michelangelo's Sonnets' (2002 reprint: p. 61):

Now that I need men's pity and compassion,
And can no longer laugh and scoff at all
The faults of others, now my soul must fall
Unguided, lacking its own domination.

Only one flag can I now serve beneath,
And with it conquer life. I speak of faith.
Only with this can I face the attack
Of all my foes, when other help I lack.

Oh flesh, Oh blood, Oh wood, Oh pain extreme!
Let all my sins be purified through you
From whom I came, as did my father too.

So good you are, your pity is supreme;
Only your help can save my evil fate:
So close to death, so far from God my state.

John Clare (1793–1864) in his poem 'I Am' (2003 reprint: p. 282) expresses his sense of desolation and separation from others in an earnest and irremediably sad voice. It is as if the poem is able to transmit to us, so that we physically experience it, the weariness and oppression in Clare's heart and how irrevocable he feels his fate to be. In this one poem we feel the power of poetry to communicate distress and despair:

I am – yet what I am, none cares or knows;
My friends forsake me like a memory lost:
I am the self-consumer of my woes –
They rise and vanish in oblivion's host
Like shadows in love-frenzied stifled throes –
And yet I am and live – like vapours tossed

Into the nothingness of scorn and noise,
Into the waking sea of living dreams
Where there is neither sense of life or joys
But the vast shipwreck of my life's esteems;
Even the dearest that I love the best
Are strange – nay, rather, stranger than the rest.

I long for scenes where man hath never trod,
A place woman never smiled or wept,
There to abide with my Creator, God,
And sleep as I in childhood sweetly slept,
Untroubling and untroubled where I lie,
The grass below – above, the vaulted sky.

Conclusion

Poetry is especially suited to expressing and describing emotional distress. In this chapter we have seen poets who have themselves experienced emotional disorders describe clinical in-patient settings, the administrative rituals of psychiatry, and the nature of the phenomena of melancholia and despair. What comes through most of all is the terrible toll of emotional disorder on the individual.

References

Berryman, J. (1989) *Collected Poems 1937–1971*. Faber and Faber Ltd.
Burnside, J. (2006a) *Selected Poems*. Jonathan Cape.
Burnside, J. (2006b) *A Lie about My Father*. Jonathan Cape.
Clare, J. (2003) *Selected Poems* (ed. J. Bate). Farrar, Strauss and Giroux LLC.
Eliot, T. S. (1957) *On Poetry and Poets*. Faber and Faber Ltd.

Gurney, I. (1982) *Collected Poems* (ed. P. J. Kavanagh). Carcanet Press.

Jennings, E. (2002) *New Collected Poems*. Carcanet Press.

Lowell, R. (1975) *Day by Day*. Farrar, Strauss and Giroux LLC.

Sexton, A. (1988) *The Selected Poems of Anne Sexton* (eds D. W. Middlebrook & D. H. George). Virago Press.

Smith, S. (1975) *Selected Poems*. Penguin Books.

Valéry, P. (1950) *Selected Writings of Paul Valéry*. New Directions Publishing.

CHAPTER 6

Letters and psychiatry: the case of Franz Kafka

Femi Oyebode

Franz Kafka (1883–1924) was born in Prague to a middle-class Jewish family. He studied law at the German Charles-Ferdinand University, graduating as a Doctor of Law in 1906. He worked as clerk for the Worker's Insurance Institute, Kingdom of Bohemia, from 1908 onwards. During this period he also continued writing. In his lifetime only his novella *The Metamorphosis* was published (in 1915). *The Trial* and *The Castle* were published posthumously (in 1925 and 1926). Kafka wrote *Letter to Father* in 1919. His father Hermann Kafka never received the letter. Extracts were published in Max Brod's biography of Franz Kafka in 1937, but the letter did not appear in its entirety until 1953, as part of the collected works of Franz Kafka.

In this chapter, *Letter to Father* will be discussed as illustration of what letters can add to an understanding of character, motivation, self-ascription and relationships. Kafka's letters to Felice Bauer (his fiancée), Ottla (his sister) and Milena Jesenskà (with whom he had a brief relationship) have also all been published. In setting the context, it is perhaps worthwhile to explore whether there is merit in studying letters of literary figures and, if there is merit in this pursuit, in what way it is constituted. There is a body of opinion that argues that the biography of a literary figure adds little to an understanding of their works. The argument here is that literary texts can only be understood in their own terms. To seek clarification from without the text is to misunderstand the purpose and methods of literature. Even an author like Paul Valéry, who accepts that extraneous influences on literature exist, is loath to accept that biography as we understand it is significant:

> The thing that is most important – the very act of the Muses – is independent of adventures, the poet's way of life, incidents, and everything that might figure in a biography. Everything that history is able to observe is insignificant.
> What is essential to the work is all the indefinable circumstances, the occult encounters, the facts that are apparent to one person alone, or so familiar to the one person that he is not even aware of them. One knows from one's experience that these incessant and impalpable events are the solid matter of one's personality [Valéry, 1950: p. 141].

Valéry appears to be saying that incidents and readily identifiable biographical details are irrelevant to understanding literature but those intrinsic aspects of personality, the fabric of the self that goes unremarked upon, are what is significant. This approach suggests that the intimate revelations in letters may signal something of importance here. But Valéry hints at a deeper problem. He argues that the self of a great writer is absolutely no one:

> How then are we to conceive the creator of a great work? But he is absolutely *no one*. How define the *Self* if it changes opinion and sides so often in the course of my work that the work is distorted under my hands; if each correction can bring about immense modifications; and if a thousand accidents of memory, attention, sensation that cross my mind appear, finally, in my finished work to be the essential ideas and original objects of my efforts? And yet it is all certainly a part of me, since my weaknesses, my strengths, my lazy repetitions, my manias, my darkness and my light, can always be recognised in everything that falls from my hands [p. 142].

This idea of the writer in the process of writing being an absence of personality is also evoked by Jorge Luis Borges in his characterisation of Shakespeare:

> There was no one in him; behind his face (which even through the bad paintings of those times resembles no other) and his words, which were copious, fantastic and stormy, there was only a bit of coldness, a dream dreamt by no one. At first he thought that all people were like him, but the astonishment of a friend to whom he had begun to speak of his emptiness showed him his error and made him feel always that an individual should not differ in outward appearance [Borges, 1964a: p. 284].

> No one has ever been so many men as this man who like the Egyptian Proteus could exhaust all the guises of reality [p. 285].

> History adds that before or after dying he found himself in the presence of God and told him: 'I who have been so many men in vain want to be one and myself.' The voice of the Lord answered from a whirlwind: 'Neither am I anyone; I have dreamt the world as you dreamt your work, my Shakespeare, and among the forms in my dream are you, who like myself are many and no one' [p. 284].

My thesis is that letters by literary figures, at least, give an insight into the character of writers. It may be that it is arguable whether letters add anything to our understanding of literary texts. But my view is that letters probably do cast a light on the psychology of writers and that the literary works of writers can be better illuminated by a study of letters. I aim to demonstrate that this is the case for Kafka.

There is an additional theoretical issue to examine at the outset. Foucault in his essay 'What is an author?' draws attention to the valorisation of an author's biography and remarks that the 'moment when the stories of heroes gave way to an author's biography; the conditions that fostered the formulation of the fundamental critical category of "the man and his work"' came about (Foucault, 1977: p. 115). The idea at stake here is that a singular relationship exists between the text and the author, particularly in the way the text points in the direction of the author, 'a figure who is outside and precedes it' (Foucault, 1977: p. 115). There is a paradox here. The author is conspicuous by his absence in the text but he none the less pervades the text. Quite often, his voice makes him readily recognisable. In a letter as opposed to fictional text, the author is ever present and his identity is what gives the letter a special quality. Thus, the letter is not merely pointing at the author but is stamped with what we take to be the authentic voice of the author. For Foucault, a private letter cannot have an author, rather it has a signatory. In this scheme, the 'function of an author is to characterize the existence, circulation, and operation of certain discourses within a society' (p. 124) and letters lie outside the boundaries of this discourse. I argue the reverse: that Kafka's *Letter to Father* is both a letter by a signatory and a literary text with an author.

Self-ascription

Kafka in this letter counterposes himself against his image of his father in order to draw a self-portrait:

> Compare the two of us: I, to put it very briefly, a Löwy with a certain Kafka foundation that, however, just isn't set in motion by the Kafka will to life, business and conquest, but by a Löwy spur that operates more secretively, more timidly, and in a different direction, and which often fails to work at all. You, on the other hand, a true Kafka in strength, health, appetite, loudness of voice, eloquence, self-satisfaction, worldly superiority, stamina, presence of mind, knowledge of human nature, a certain generosity; of course, also with all the failings and weaknesses that go with these advantages, into which your temperament and sometimes your violent temper drive you [Kafka, 1999 reprint: p. 12].

There is dispute about whether this self-characterisation is an accurate representation of Kafka. It may simply be a rhetorical device that allowed Kafka to describe his father. There is no doubt that the descriptive terms he uses to characterise his father start as positive but the final sentence has a sting in its tail: 'of course, with all the failings and weaknesses that go with these advantages'. Kafka's self-description includes his perception of his physique compared with that of his father:

> I was skinny, weakly, slight; you were strong, tall, broad. Even in the changing-room I felt pitiful, and what's more, not only in your eyes, but in the eyes of the entire world, for you were for me the standard by which everything was measured ... I was grateful to you that you did not appear to notice my anguish; I was proud, too, of my father's body [p. 16].

In these self-definitions, Kafka is using a literary device of making sharply delineated and contrasting portraits, amplified by exaggerations of features. The exaggerative effects are achieved by creating a superfluity of adjectives that causes a pictorial distance between two objects. In another section, Kafka compares himself with his sister Valli, better known as Elli:

> She was such a clumsy, tired, timid, morose, guilt-ridden, overly humble, malicious, lazy, greedy, stingy child I could hardly look at her; certainly not speak to her, *so much did she remind me of myself* [my italics], so very similarly was she under the same spell of our upbringing [p. 38].

In this extract, Kafka identifies himself with Valli's faults, as if sharing particular characteristics with someone else might somehow render the force of these failings less pernicious. The negative attributes are primarily Valli's, although of course shared by Kafka. The passage also hints at Kafka's sense of unworthiness. This attaches to his view of his own body, as already described above, but also links his bodily dissatisfaction with a preoccupation with his physical health:

> I became unsure of even the things nearest to me, my own body. I grew very tall but didn't know what to do with my height, the burden was too great, my back became bent; I hardly dared to move, let alone exercise, I remained weak; I regarded everything I still had at my command as a miracle, for instance my good digestion; that sufficed to lose it, and even with that the way was open to every form of hypochondria until finally, under the superhuman effort of wanting to marry ... blood came from the lungs [p. 53].

This preoccupation with his physical habitus is expressed in his exchange of letters with Felice Bauer, to whom he was engaged for a period. His physique was linked, at least in his mind, with his literary style: 'Just as I am thin, and I am the thinnest person I know (and that's saying something, for I am no stranger to sanatoria), there is also nothing to me which, in relation to writing one could call superfluous, superfluous in the sense of overflowing' (Kafka, 1967 reprint: p. 120).

Kafka's expressed low self-esteem often strikes one as a pose, a mannerism that either unconsciously or deliberately masks a determined and incisive spirit, a spirit far from the weak and effete portrait that Kafka liked to project. In a letter to Felice dated 16 June 1913, he wrote:

> I am nothing, absolutely nothing. I am 'further ahead in every way' than you? Some capacity for understanding people, and for putting myself in their place – this I have, but I don't believe that I have ever met a single person who in the long run in his ordinary human relationships, in normal everyday life (and what else is it all about?), could be more hopeless than I. I have no memory, either of things learned or things heard, either of people or events: I feel as though I had experienced nothing, learned nothing, and in fact I know less about most things than the average schoolboy; and what I know, I know so superficially that even the second question is beyond me. I am unable to reason, my reasoning constantly comes up against a blank wall; certain isolated facts I can grasp in a flash, but I am quite incapable of coherent, consecutive reasoning. *Nor can I tell a story properly* [my italics]; in fact I can hardly even talk [1967 reprint: p. 388].

In this extract, does Kafka actually believe what he asserts? Is this a method, a stratagem for seeking the approval of Felice Bauer, so that her response can affirm the positive about him? Or is it the case that Kafka does not believe in himself? So far we have seen Kafka unfavourably compare himself with his father and liken himself to his sister Valli, in her negative aspects. In relation to Felice Bauer, he also casts a negative light on himself and uses this as the basis for not proceeding towards marriage:

> Now consider, Felice, the change that marriage would bring about for us, what each would lose and each would gain. I should lose my (for the most part) terrible loneliness, and you, whom I love above all others, would be my gain. Whereas you would lose the life you have lived hitherto, with which you were almost completely satisfied. You would lose Berlin, the office you enjoy, your girlfriends, the small pleasures of life, the prospect of marrying a decent, cheerful, healthy man, of having beautiful, healthy children for whom, if you think about it, you clearly long. In place of these incalculable losses, you would gain a sick, weak, unsociable, taciturn, gloomy, stiff, almost hopeless man who possibly has but one virtue, which is that he loves you. Instead of sacrificing yourself for real children, which would be in accordance with your nature as a healthy girl, you would have to sacrifice yourself for this man who is childish, but childish in the worst sense, and who at best can learn from you, letter by letter, the ways of human speech [p. 390].

In *Letter to Father*, Kafka gives different reasons for not proceeding from engagement to marriage. His explanations call on the troubled relationship with his father rather than on the disadvantages to Felice Bauer of marrying a person such as himself. Of course, human conduct is often overdetermined. Multiple layers of meaning and motivation drive behaviour. And it is perfectly plausible that both excuses were true. In psychology there need not be a logic that says that one cause excludes all others. Kafka argues that as his parents' marriage was successful, marrying was a territory that his father already occupied and that this territory was therefore denied to him. The language is graphic:

> But being as we are, marrying is barred to me because it is your very own territory. Sometimes I imagine the map of the world spread out and you stretched out diagonally across it. And then it seems to me as though I could consider living in those places that you either do not cover or that do not lie within your reach. And, in keeping with the conception that I have of your size, these are not many and not very comforting regions, and especially marriage is not among them [Kafka, 1999 reprint: p. 65].

Kafka goes on to argue that his lofty idea of marriage was formed on the model of his parents' marriage. He denies that his aversion to marriage was due to the 'fear that one's children would some day pay one back for the sins committed against one's own parents' (p. 65). He concludes that there is anxiety about him that emanates from his desire for independence, to 'escape with the smallest success' (p. 66). Marriage posits the merest possibility that his independence would be compromised and thus he renounced it. This explanation is closer to the truth in my view. It is searching and close to the bone. It acknowledges Kafka's need for independence, his reluctance to be moored by a spouse, no matter how supportive the partnership might be. In another sense it locates his renunciation of marriage within his drive for success as a writer. There were ancillary stirrings that put him off marriage:

recognition that his parents' successful marriage required something that he had seen in his father, namely his father's strength, which he was not convinced he himself possessed.

Significantly in the following passage in *Letter to Father*, Kafka made explicit the multidimensional nature of his father's character. We start to see a more complex portrait of the man; not a cardboard cut-out figure, whose sole role was as a mirror to reflect aspects of Kafka that he thought either undesirable or worthy:

> Strength and the mocking of others, health and a certain excessiveness, eloquence and inadequacy, self-confidence and dissatisfaction with everyone else, worldly sovereignty and tyranny, knowledge of human nature and mistrust of most, then also good points without any drawbacks, such as diligence, endurance, presence of mind and fearlessness. By comparison, I had almost nothing of all this or only very little, and on this basis I dared to want to marry when I saw for myself that *even you* [my italics] had to struggle hard in marriage and where the children were concerned, even failed? [p. 69].

Roots

Kafka's self-portrait is akin to an extended account of personality within a clinical encounter. It employs all the devices for self-characterisation: contrast with the other; identification with the other; and exaggeration that requires modifying response. What it lacks is the objectifying view of the other, the traditional response to the question 'How do others see you?'. By definition, a letter is addressed to another person, therefore reading Kafka's letter is like eavesdropping on a personal and intimate conversation between two people. This distinguishes letters from other kinds of narrative, such as autobiography and fiction. Autobiography and fiction are written for public consumption, whereas letters, like diaries, are primarily intended for scrutiny in private. This fact alone makes both letters and diaries worthy of the interest of psychiatrists. It may be possible within this space of the private and personal to derive some understanding of what motivates human behaviour, at least in the sense in which it is understood by the protagonists themselves. There is merit also in the understanding that individuals reach about their own situation which is unsullied by the doctrinaire conceptions of modern psychiatry as often dictated by the various schools of the dynamic unconscious.

In *Letter to Father*, Kafka renders a view about what the singular event was that determined a significant aspect of himself:

> One night I kept on whimpering for water, certainly not because I was thirsty, but probably partly to be annoying, partly to amuse myself. After several strong threats had not helped, you took me out of bed, carried me out onto the pavlatche and left me standing there alone for a little while in my nightshirt outside the locked door. I do not want to say that this was wrong, perhaps there was really no other way at the time to acquire peace and quiet that night, but I only want to characterize by this your child-rearing methods

and their effect on me. After that I was really quite obedient, but I came away from it with *internal damage* [my italics]. What was for me self-evident, my pointless asking for water, and the extreme terror of being carried outside were two things that I, my nature being what it was, could never properly connect. Even years afterward I still suffered from the tormenting fancy that that enormous man, my father, the ultimate authority, could for almost no reason come during the night and take me out of bed and carry me out onto the pavlatche, and that meant that *I was a mere nothing to him* [my italics; p. 14].

This singular event, at least from Kafka's point of view, played a role in creating in him 'this feeling of nothingness that often overwhelms' (p. 14). Now whether this event and others like it should bear the burden of Kafka's self-portrait is a moot point. It is possible that Kafka, recognising in himself particular attitudes, might have in his search for self-understanding come to lay the blame on events such as the one described above. Kafka is aware of this possibility. Although he is obviously blaming his father for much of the weaknesses that he perceives in himself, he is also conscious that this is a treacherous position to take: 'I am not saying that I have become what I am only as a result of your influence. That would be very much an exaggeration (and, in fact, *I lean towards this exaggeration*)' (my italics; p. 11). Furthermore, he says 'I would probably have become a shy and anxious person in any case, but it is still a long, dark road from there to where I have really come' (p. 43). But, on balance, Kafka leans towards the belief that the events that he records are at the root of his personal difficulties.

Kafka recounts how his father brought up the children by means of irony but also spoke to them through their mother:

> Provocative were also those rebukes in which one was treated as a third person, not even considered worthy of being angrily addressed; when you speak formally to Mother, but actually to me, who was sitting right there, for example: 'Of course, that is too much to expect of our worthy son,' and the like. (This produced a corollary in that, for example, I didn't dare to ask you directly, and later, out of habit, didn't even think of asking you directly when Mother was around. It was much less dangerous for the child to put a question about you to Mother, sitting beside you; one asked Mother then: 'How is Father?' and thus protected oneself against surprises.) [pp. 26–27].

For Kafka, this produced 'a sullen, inattentive, disobedient child, always on the run, mainly within himself' (p. 27). And we can see his reasoning, a tyrannical father who is both physically big and emotionally autocratic, terrorises the child into passivity and taciturnity. The facts apparently speak against this. Many commentators have said that Kafka was neither passive nor taciturn. In fact, Anz (1999) argues that in *Letter to Father*, Kafka used many of the same literary devices that he employed in his fictional works and that his tendency to exaggeration was prominent in the *Letter*. Also, the *Letter* draws on the same themes as in Kafka's fiction: anxiety and guilt, accusations and condemnation, freedom and power, artistry and profession, and so on. Anz further argues that an authentic portrait of Kafka's personality and autobiography cannot be gained from reading *Letter to Father* (Anz, 1999). This latter point seems extreme. It is true that Kafka's father never received the letter. It is thought that it started out as a short letter but very quickly developed into 100 pages of handwritten text. It reads like a literary work but was undoubtedly written with a particular audience in mind, namely his father. The self-portrayals, even if exaggerated, ring true. The self-understanding is transparent. The discussions about the possible roots of his difficulties also are plausible. But, as with all human documents of this kind, there are hints of self-deception, of the desire to accuse others, to score points, to influence opinion and to project particular aspects of the self for effect. None of these very human predilections argues against employing the *Letter* as a basis for understanding Kafka and for approaching his fiction with a view to greater clarity. The trick is to be aware of the limitations of this method.

Understanding the works

My intention is not to undertake a major examination of Kafka's literary corpus on the basis of my reading of *Letter to Father*. Rather, it is to ask whether there is merit in making such an investigation. The subtext is: can understanding a person assist us in understanding their performances, that is, their literary works, in adult life? I mean by this, whether understanding personal motivation can inform how people behave, including the content of their writings or how they manage their businesses, etc. In a sense this question can be answered only in the affirmative. Literary works, like all other products of the human psyche, are subject to the same laws: a writer's preoccupations are reflections of their inner life, which are in turn manifestations of their experiences. None the less, for psychiatrists, demonstrating this is itself interesting and informative. It could explicitly demonstrate how these relationships are manifested. There is an additional subtext: how do we read a person so that we come to know them enough to understand their motivations? It is claimed that a study of literary texts allows us to privilege language: this in turn means that we come to see how to attend to language, the multiple possibilities of meaning; the hidden and the overt; the missing information and the red herring that acts as decoy; the varied and rich methods people use in communicating not only distress but love and hostility. And all the things that are unsaid but which are real and influence behaviour and emotions.

Elias Canetti (1974) in *Kafka's Other Trial* wrote: 'Kafka is, of all writers, the greatest expert in power. He has experienced and shaped it in each of its aspects' (p. 62). This notion that Kafka's writings deal with power relations is a good starting point. We have seen how in his letters he drew a sharp comparison between himself and his father; how in this comparison he identified the differences in physical size and strength, and also in drive and passion. He refers to the tyranny of his father; his father's authority not only within the home but also at work. In his novella *The Metamorphosis* (1915), Kafka wrote a story about a man who wakes one morning to find himself transformed into a dung beetle. The story can be read at several levels. It is the case that in reading any novel, care must be taken about any possible interpretations. Borges (1964*b*) once wrote 'every writer *creates* his own precursors. His work modifies our conception of the past, as it will modify the future' (p. 236). Although here Borges was referring to how, once we come upon Kafka's work, we can see how other writers gave birth to him as we can what other writers he gave birth to. The question of derivation is fraught with problems. This is also true for how we might see in Kafka's own novels precursors from his letters and biography. The point is that these associations and conceptions of derivation are illusory and represent points of similarity rather than of origin. None the less, it is noteworthy that in *The Metamorphosis*, the story is set within a family that could be any family, but that appears familiar to us in its composition and functioning. If we know Kafka's family life, in reading *The Metamorphosis* we feel as if once again we are before Kafka's family. Our protagonist is named Gregor Samsa; it is perhaps not without significance that the name 'Samsa' has onomatopoeic characteristics similar to those of 'Kafka'. This suggests that Gregor Samsa may be readily identified with Kafka. There are straightforward differences in the cast: Samsa works to keep his family, including his father, whereas Kafka's father was an industrious and energetic man. Even this difference can be understood as the symmetrical opposite of Kafka's own family. But, the emotions enacted within the plot are understandable in the light of what we know about the Kafka household. The father becomes aggressive and assaultive; the mother is passive but well-meaning; and the sister is initially very supportive and has a special relationship with Gregor Samsa. The emotional tone that pervades the story – guilt, shame, feelings of oppression and entrapment, unworthiness and low self-esteem – is recognisable from what we know about Kafka's own life within his family. Kafka's letters do not hold the key to understanding *The Metamorphosis*. The novella can be read without recourse to the letters. But, in my view, there is a deepening of understanding, a clarity about the landscape of the emotions in the story, that is absent without having read the letters. It is as if the novels are part of Kafka's life rather than independent appendages that have a life all of their own. This suggests that the literary works continue as extensions of the author, that they are means of understanding the person. It may be that the creative works are actually means by which an author explores their own life and that properly decoded they give an entry into the personal and private, even the secretive aspect of the author's life. This conclusion is in opposition to the idea that fiction can only be understood in its own terms and that it points nowhere but to the hermeneutics of the plot. It is a surprising conclusion; the literary works deepen our understanding of the author, for they are extensions of the author's emotional life.

Conclusion

Letters are unique communications. They are different from autobiography and fiction in that they are addressed to a known and identifiable individual. Their content can be mundane or intimate. They can be more directly revealing of the nature of relationships. And as we have seen, they can add to our knowledge of an author's life. I believe too that they may help illuminate the works of creative writers. For psychiatrists, they add to our understanding of how emotional life thrives and influences behaviour and creative works. In Kafka's case, they are supremely valuable in revealing how language works to express anger and envy, how it cherishes unworthiness as a prize, how it accuses yet consoles, and how it can masquerade as diffidence and modesty while being eloquent and wounding. But, most urgently, the letters show how important it is to attend to language, and psychiatry is nothing if not a subject enacted within language.

References

Anz, T. (1999) Afterword. In *Letter to Father* (trans. K Reppin). Vitalis.

Borges, J. L. (1964a) Everything and nothing. In *Labyrinths: Selected Stories and Other Writings* (eds D. A. Yates & J. E. Irby), pp. 284–285. Penguin Books.

Borges, J. L. (1964b) Kafka and his precursors. In *Labyrinths: Selected Stories and Other Writings* (eds D. A. Yates & J. E. Irby), pp. 234–236). Penguin Books.

Brod, M. (1937) *Franz Kafka, eine Biographie*. Reprinted (1974) as *Franz Kafka, a Biography*. Da Capo Press.

Canetti, E. (1974) *Kafka's Other Trial: The Letters to Felice* (trans. C Middleton). Penguin Books.

Foucault, M. (1977) What is an author? In *Language, Counter-Memory, Practice: Selected Essays and Interviews* (ed. D. F. Bouchard, trans. D. F. Bouchard & S. Simon), pp. 113–138.

Kafka, F. (1919) *Brief an den Vater*. Reprinted (1999) as *Letter to Father* (trans. K Reppin). Vitalis.

Kafka F. (1912–1917) *Letters to Felice*. Reprinted (1967): eds E. Heller & J. Born, trans. J. Stern & E. Duckworth. Penguin Books.

Kafka F. (1915) *Die Verwandlung*. Reprinted (1946) as The Metamorphosis, in *The Complete Stories* (ed. N. N. Glatzer), pp. 89–139. Schocken Books.

Valéry, P. (1950) *The Selected Writings of Paul Valéry*. New Directions Publishing.

CHAPTER 7

Death and dying in literature

John Skelton

How do people write about death and dying? At one end of the scale there are the sometimes embarrassing but often deeply personal and profoundly felt lines of doggerel on tombstones or in the 'In memoriam' columns of newspapers ('She faltered by the wayside and the angels took her home'). The internet is a great source of bathetic epitaphs, many no doubt apocryphal. At the other end of the scale, there is death in great literature, for example King Lear's lament over his dead daughter Cordelia. This extraordinary scene concludes:

> No, no, no life!
> Why should a dog, a horse, a rat, have life,
> And thou no breath at all? Thou'lt come no more,
> Never, never, never, never, never!
> Pray you, undo this button: thank you, sir.
> Do you see this? Look on her, look, her lips,
> Look there, look there!

(King Lear: Act V, scene iii)

And Lear himself dies, perhaps under the delusion that Cordelia still lives, an audience's desire for a happy ending ambiguously usurped by Shakespeare. The play was reworked, in fact, in the 18th century with a happy ending grafted on to reflect the more optimistic ethos of the age. And in our own time, Edward Bond wrote a version of the Lear story (Bond, 1972) which was bleaker than Shakespeare's original, precisely on the grounds that Shakespeare was too optimistic. One of the central things of which literature can make us more aware is that death means different things at different times.

But these two kinds of text – the banal and the sublime – clearly have things in common. They attempt, for example, to express bereavement and give shape to our thoughts about death. The first affirms a belief in the final, Christian, order of the universe; and it is the question of order that Shakespeare, too, addresses: Where is justice if the good die young?

The simplest truth about great literature – 'Literature' with a capital 'L' – is that it makes use of death for its own purposes. The death of Cordelia, however moving we may find it on stage, is among other things, and perhaps some would want to argue principally, a functional device. Shakespeare writes the scene, of course, to bring home to us the awfulness of death: but also to bring together the themes of the play: the world's injustice, the death of innocence, Lear's final recognition of his own foolishness, and so on. And in fact though the death of Cordelia, in a good production, can be overwhelmingly powerful, many fictional deaths are not really intended to be terribly moving. They may be plot devices to remove someone from the scene, or produce a glow of satisfaction in the reader that someone has got their just deserts, and so on. The victims in murder stories, to take the simplest example, are usually just pieces of the puzzle. And indeed one of the set-piece scenes of the thriller – the description of violent death (a kind of set piece not always designed to give us greater insight into the nature of death, or the horror of violence, or the motivation of the psychologically disturbed) is played beautifully in Nabokov's *Lolita* (Nabokov, 1955), a book that subverts much more than our notions of acceptable sexual behaviour. Here, the protagonist kills his nemesis, Clare Quilty, whom Lolita, the teenage object of obsession, has preferred to him:

> Suddenly dignified, and somewhat morose, he started to walk up the broad stairs, and, shifting my position, but not actually following him up the steps, I fired three or four times in quick succession, wounding him at every blaze; and every time I did it to him, that horrible thing to him, his face would twitch in an absurd clownish manner, as if he were exaggerating the pain; he slowed down, rolled his eyes half closing them and made a feminine 'ah!' and he shivered every time a bullet hit him as if I were tickling him, and every time I got him with those slow, clumsy, blind bullets of mine, he would say under his breath, with a phony British accent – all the while dreadfully twitching, shivering, smirking, but withal talking in a curiously detached and even amiable manner: 'Ah, that hurts, sir, enough! Ah, that hurts atrociously, my dear fellow. I pray you, desist. Ah – very painful, very painful, indeed … God! Hah! This is abominable, you should really not – ' His voice trailed off as he reached the landing, but he steadily walked on despite all the lead I had lodged in his bloated body – and in distress, in dismay, I understood that far from killing him I was injecting spurts of energy into the poor fellow, as if the bullets had been capsules wherein a heady elixir danced.
>
> I reloaded the thing with hands that were black and bloody – I had touched something he had anointed with his thick gore. Then I rejoined him upstairs, the keys jangling in my pockets like gold.
>
> He was trudging from room to room, bleeding majestically, trying to find an open window, shaking his head, and still trying to talk me out of murder. I took aim at his head, and he retired to the master bedroom with a burst of royal purple where his ear had been [1995 reprint, pp. 301–302].

(In fact, as we learn, the truth is that Lolita has preferred Quilty utterly: the sudden, devastating comparison of the two both makes this clear and reveals the seriousness of the novel beneath the gloriously inventive word-spinning: 'He broke my heart: you merely broke my life' (p. 277)).

In other words, literature is not just an attack on the emotions: and even where the emotions are involved, it may not be a sense of grief that is elicited. It is not always the aim of literature to present us with death in such a way as to make us feel personally bereaved: and in great literature, though a sense of bereavement may be the starting point for our own reveries about what we have seen or read, the aim is never merely the bereavement. Rather, it is the broader issue of what the death means.

Nor, on the other hand, is it only great literature that expresses emotions.

Personal accounts

The power of the arts and of artifice is ambivalent. It can blind the reader to sentimental trash. Who has not cried at the death of Bambi's mother? How many of us have tuned into a favourite soap (in an earlier age, a 'weepie', as such melodramas of the silver screen were known) with a box of tissues in one hand, a box of chocolates in the other, and allowed a sense of luxurious sadness to consume us? Which girl – it seems only girls read it – has not wept over the demise of Beth in Louisa M. Alcott's *Little Women* (Alcott, 1868)?

Dickens is the litmus test here. Unquestionably a great writer, yet prey to what we think of as the excesses of a sentimental age. Here, he describes the death of the impoverished child, Little Nell, in *The Old Curiosity Shop* (Dickens, 1840–41). (Dickens owed an immediate debt to Shakespeare in his work: indeed, it is a measure of his greatness that he has the confidence to borrow from him, and so openly risk comparison. Note the similarities between this death and that of Cordelia, above). The first speaker is the old man whom Nell has befriended:

> 'She is still asleep,' he whispered. 'You were right. She did not call – unless she did so in her slumber.'
>
> 'She has called to me in her sleep before now, Sir; as I have sat by, watching, I have seen her lips move, and have known, though no sound came from them, that she spoke of me. I feared the light might dazzle her eyes and wake her, so I brought it here...'
>
> '...She is sleeping soundly,' he said; 'but no wonder. Angel hands have strewn the ground deep with snow, that the lightest footstep may be lighter yet; and the very birds are dead, that they may not wake her. She used to feed them, Sir. Though never so cold and hungry, the timid things would fly from us. They never flew from her!' [Dickens, 2001 reprint: pp. 534–535].

But, like Lear, the old man is mistaken:

> For she was dead. There, upon her little bed, she lay at rest. The solemn stillness was no marvel now.
>
> She was dead. No sleep so beautiful and calm, so free from trace of pain, so fair to look upon. She seemed a creature fresh from the hand of God, and waiting for the breath of life; not one who had lived and suffered death.
>
> Her couch was dressed with here and there some winter berries and green leaves, gathered in a spot she had been used to favour. 'When I die, put near me something that has loved the light, and had the sky above it always.' Those were her words.
>
> ... She was dead. Dear, gentle, patient, noble Nell was dead...

And still her former self lay there, unaltered in this change. Yes. The old fireside had smiled upon that same sweet face; it had passed, like a dream, through haunts of misery and care; at the door of the poor schoolmaster on the summer evening, before the furnace fire upon the cold wet night, at the still bedside of the dying boy, there had been the same mild lovely look. So shall we know the angels in their majesty, after death [p. 540].

If this does not move us to abject surrender and sentimental tears, the emotions evoked might be more complex and less forgiving. As Oscar Wilde once remarked, 'One must have a heart of stone to read the death of little Nell without laughing' (Pearson, 1946: p. 208). Perhaps. A complex mix of embarrassment, humour and dismay colours our response to both this and amateur verse, or the attempts of the poorly equipped to strike a formal note of gravity.

This does not mean that poverty of expression is the same as poverty of feeling. One of the lessons of King Lear, after all, is that true feelings lie too deep for words: beware those who, like Lear's wicked daughters, can articulate their love. Trust rather the saintly Cordelia, the daughter whose love is deep beyond expression. By extension, for just this reason a dying patient or a bereaved relative may welcome the release that literature brings. They may feel that their own power to express themselves has failed and that there is relief in the words of others and the possibility of saying 'This is what I mean'.

This makes for an ambivalence in much of the writing about death and dying. Sometimes it is profoundly felt, sometimes it is profoundly expressed, but not often is it both. Here is an example from a website (www.familyfriendpoems.com/family/death-poems.asp):

So many things we never got to do
So many conversations we never got through
I feel lost and empty now
Every day I ask, how?

…and so on. Halting verse, technically naïve, vacuous sentiment: yet perfectly real, perfectly honest in a way that some very highly regarded writers do not manage.

Then, placed between the great writer and the amateur versifier are the articulate, contemporary professionals, often with accounts of their own illness, their own forthcoming demise, by people who have made a living out of words. Often, as with John Diamond (1999) and Oscar Moore (1996), journalists who were victims of throat cancer and AIDS respectively, an easy sophistication hangs over their work. But this is a game whose rules many of us understand, and the writing has an immediate power, closely linked to our confidence that we know what is going on. This is Moore, talking about going blind:

Dwindling in weight and morale, I fled to out-of-town friends and spent two days sitting in a garden on Long Island recuperating … i.e. napping. So it should have been easy to blame my foggy vision and guerrilla headbangs on a combination of red-eye flight and nap overdose. Unfortunately not.

You see (I hate sight verbs!) the fog wasn't unseasonal bonfires or post-night-flight blur, and the headaches weren't random flares. We were at war, and losing it. The CMV had woken up with a hunger, and I now had so little retina left on the left that my vision was getting to be like US television – hardly enough pixels to make a picture [Moore, 1996: p. 166].

The writing is self-consciously able and literate. Moore effortlessly strings his war metaphors together, for example. Is it 'good writing'? Well, that depends what you want from it, perhaps. It is clever, the emotions all mediated through a somewhat distancing intelligence. It is techni-cally adept: it is approachable, and for all the quizzical distance the author maintains from his condition, it has a kind of immediacy. There is urgency, captured in the compound adjectives ('out-of-town', 'red-eye', 'post-night-flight'), the throwaway stylistic trick of a man accustomed to make words work for him. The prose has the kind of easy self-regarding commentary ('I hate sight verbs!') that looks cool, ironic, post-modern. But is it hon-est, beneath the showy intelligence? Perhaps the answer is merely that the illness is real enough, after all. And that this book, and similar accounts, have given a sense of authenticity to readers, and perhaps also a sense of a shared plight to some. In the end, you might want to argue, it is not for the quality of his thoughts or feelings that we read this, but for the sense of the person which shines through. In that respect, it matters less what is said than who says it.

Making sense of death

One of the central tasks of literature is to impose a structure on life and death, giving meaning to both. Indeed, literature as a discipline aims just as certainly as science does to understand the world in which we live and to interpret our own role as participants in the human condition. The dif-ficulty for the non-specialist is understanding the various ways in which literature works: this is particularly true when it comes to the question of understanding across time and space.

Here is one example, which is fairly well-known and relatively approachable. And – much more so than is the case with Moore, whose well-honed literary talents are not really so very rare – this is by Tennyson and therefore the work of a master technician, a craftsman with a better ear for the effects poetry can create through sound than almost anyone else, certainly in English. Perhaps the poem also corresponds to a certain rather old-fashioned idea of what poetry is in its effortless rhythmical dexterity:

Dark house, by which once more I stand
Here in the long unlovely street,
Doors, where my heart was used to beat
So quickly, waiting for a hand,

A hand that can be clasp'd no more –
Behold me, for I cannot sleep,
And like a guilty thing I creep
At earliest morning to the door.

He is not here; but far away
The noise of life begins again,
And ghastly thro' the drizzling rain
On the bald street breaks the blank day.

(Tennyson, *In Memoriam*, VII)

Tennyson's 'In Memoriam', from which this is taken, is a long – very long – series of short poems (published in 1849) following the death of his close friend, Arthur Hallam. Hallam was a brilliant young man (just 22 when he died), and it seems clear that Tennyson expected to spend the rest of his life in close contact with him. The deeply felt grief makes it a personal account, but deep feeling refined into literature. Note, in particular, a much-quoted example of Tennyson's genius in the way that the easy, gentle sweep of the poem is hijacked in the last line by the sudden change of rhythm. It is an effect managed by a very simple trick. The typical rhythm of this poem, and of vast swathes of English poetry, is 'te-tum, te-tum'. But to say the last line with this rhythm would mean putting stress on the word 'the' on both occasions: so one ends up stressing instead the words 'bald' and 'blank'. In a sense, the poem is held together by poetic technique; the feelings behind it are so bleak that it is hard to see how they found expression at all.

Behind the sadness, hovering off-stage for much of the time in the poems of 'In Memoriam', and entirely absent in this one, is the apparatus of Victorian life and, in particular, the solace of the Christian faith. This, of course, has been the backdrop to a great deal of Western literature about death and dying. Christianity has offered a way of understanding grief and our own death in the context of eternity.

At its literary best, faith lends a power and conviction to writing which speaks clearly to those of other faiths, or none. This is John Donne (*c.* 1609), who became a cleric in later life:

Death be not proud, though some have called thee
Mighty and dreadful, for, thou art not so,
For, those, whom thou thinks't, thou dost overthrow,
Die not, poor death, nor yet canst thou kill me;
From rest and sleep, which but thy pictures be,
Much pleasure, then from thee, much more must flow,
And soonest our best men with thee do go,
Rest of their bones, and soul's delivery.
Thou art slave to fate, chance, kings and desperate men,
And dost with poison, war and sickness dwell,
And poppy, or charms can make us sleep as well,
And better than thy stroke; why swells't thou then?
One short sleep past, we wake eternally,
And death shall be no more, Death thou shalt die.'

(Donne, Holy Sonnet X: 'Death, Be Not Proud')

Here, the effect is of passion and a kind of driven commitment, one might say, reinforced by the tight verse form of the sonnet, which is handled effortlessly and compacts a great deal of meaning into a short space. This poem too is a masterpiece of technique. Like Oscar Moore's account, there is both intelligence and emotion at work here, but the intelligence, and the craftsmanship that manifests it, are entirely in the service of the feelings that drive the poem. What guarantees the value of the writing is not who is writing but what is said and how.

It also works because of the shared understanding that most readers will have of the cultural and religious context, even if they do not actually share the belief system. In other words, cultural familiarity is of substantial importance. One of the central lessons one derives from the study of literary death is how perceptions of it change through time and place.

Contrast even Donne, for example, who is several hundred years removed from us, and contrast too writing from other cultures, whose social value is now more or less entirely lost. The Ancient Egyptians set great store by the account of themselves written on their tombs, but these texts, sometimes called 'autobiographies', have no real meaning to us now, unless we are archaeologists or historians. (Then Avaris was sacked. I brought away from there as plunder one man and three women. His Majesty gave them to me as slaves... (Tyldesley, 1998)). Similarly, the following is a poem written by Basho, the great Japanese writer of haiku, as death approached. It is extremely famous, much translated (the example below is from Oseko, 1990: p. 329) and, without a knowledge of Japanese culture, fairly vacuous:

> Ill on a journey,
> My dreams still wandering round
> Over withered fields.

What do such things mean? – very little without the shared culture; without, for example, a sense of the resonance of the word 'dream' (*yume*), which pervades the short Japanese poem and has been picked up, played with and enriched by author after author over centuries.

Symbolic deaths

Clearly, much of what is quoted above is literature striving to demonstrate that particular deaths fit into some kind of overall scheme. This may be an eschatological account of the world or merely a matter of taking death seriously because we, in turn, hope that our death will be taken seriously. At any rate, what matters is the context in which death is placed. But literature itself is such that death has many functions. In other words, the context of literature gives death and dying many roles to play.

At one end of the scale is one of the most common types of death in all fiction, the discovery of the body in the 'whodunnit' or murder mystery. This may require us to expend no deeper emotion than we do on a crossword puzzle, or it may, as in the next example, aim to do more. This is from *Smiley's People* (1979) by the great novelist of the spy-story John le Carré. His hero, Smiley, has just discovered a body:

Slowly, [Smiley] returned his gaze to Leipzig's face. Some dead faces, he reflected, have the dull, even stupid look of a patient under anaesthetic. Others preserve a single mood of the once varied nature – the dead man as lover, as father, as car driver, bridge player, tyrant. And some, like Leipzig's, have ceased to preserve anything. But Leipzig's face, even without the ropes across it, had a mood, and it was anger: anger intensified by pain, turned to fury by it; anger that had increased and become the whole man as the body lost its strength [Le Carré, 2000 reprint: p. 243].

This is almost a meditation on the nature of death. However, the focus immediately changes to death as a puzzle:

Methodically, Smiley peered about him, thinking as slowly as he could manage, trying, by his examination of the debris, to reconstruct their progress. First the fight before they overpowered him, which he deduced from the smashed table-legs and chairs and lamps and shelves ... Then the search, which took place after they had trussed him and in the intervals while they had questioned him [p. 243].

One stage further on is the kind of book, often called a 'whydunnit', in which the identity of the killer is not as important as their motivation. Bear in mind here that the greatest of all constraints on the writers of whodunnits is that they cannot describe the motivations of their characters well, or it will be at once clear who is the killer. The complete blandness of Agatha Christie characters is necessary, in this respect, to fulfil the genre's requirements – or at least it is a happy accident. Contrast this with Charles Dickens' *The Mystery of Edwin Drood* (1870), which is, among other things, a whodunnit. Famously, Dickens died before revealing the identity of the killer, but it can be determined with near certainty from the imagery and symbolism with which Dickens surrounds him throughout the book.

The function of the hero's death in tragedy and epic is one of the oldest literary conventions. We have looked at King Lear but it is worth reminding ourselves of the way the idea of the good death varies from society to society. This is the death of the Trojan hero Sarpedon. Homer's text is here translated by Alexander Pope, whose urbane 18th-century style puts a neo-classical veneer on Homer's more direct original:

The towering chiefs to fiercer fight advance:
And first Sarpedon whirl'd his weighty lance,
Which o'er the warrior's shoulder took its course,
And spent in empty air its dying force.
Not so Patroclus' never-erring dart;
Aim'd at his breast it pierced a mortal part,
Where the strong fibres bind the solid heart.
Then as the mountain oak, or poplar tall,
Or pine (fit mast for some great admiral)
Nods to the axe, till with a groaning sound
It sinks, and spreads its honours on the ground,
Thus fell the king; and laid on earth supine,
Before his chariot stretch'd his form divine:
He grasp'd the dust distain'd with streaming gore,
And, pale in death, lay groaning on the shore.

So lies a bull beneath the lion's paws,
While the grim savage grinds with foamy jaws
The trembling limbs, and sucks the smoking blood;
Deep groans, and hollow roars, rebellow through the wood.

(Pope, *The Iliad of Homer*, 1715–1720)

And let us pick up the story in Christopher Logue's 20th-century version – a reworking, rather than a translation, but differing form Pope in a great deal more than that:

Air into azure steel
The daylight stiffens to translucent horn;
And through it
Falling
One sun's cord
Opening out into a radiant cone around Sarpedon's corpse;
And him inside that light, as if
A god asleep upon his outstretched hand.
.
.
.

Dust like red mist.
Pain like chalk on slate. Heat like Arctic.
The light withdrawn from Sarpedon's body.
The enemies swirling over it.
Bronze flak.

(Logue, *War Music*, 1981)

This captures what we imagine to be the vivid originality, the ferocious power, of the story as its first audiences heard it (Homer being part of the oral tradition). Perhaps in its time Pope's translation did something of the same.

The death scene in war, and the dying warrior, are conventions of Homeric verse, and of many other traditions too, just as the discovery of the body is a convention of the whodunnit. Literature is full of deaths of one sort or another, most of them offering a climax in a plot, a point of reflection, and an opportunity to take stock

The following is part of the death scene of the consumptive Ralph Touchett, in Henry James's exquisite novel *The Portrait of a Lady* (1881). When his close friend Isabel visits him, she finds at first that his face on his deathbed is, in an astonishing phrase, 'as still as the lid on a box'. Then, after some days, he is briefly well enough to talk:

'What does it matter if I'm tired when I've all eternity to rest? There's no harm in making an effort when it's the very last of all. Don't people always feel better just before the end? I've often heard of that; it's what I was waiting for. Ever since you've been here I thought it would come. I tried two or three times; I was afraid you'd get tired of sitting there.' ... 'It was very good of you to come,' he went on. 'I thought you would; but I wasn't sure.'

'I was not sure either till I came,' said Isabel.

'You've been like an angel beside my bed. You know they talk about the angel of death. It's the most beautiful of all. You've been like that; as if you were waiting for me.'

'I was not waiting for your death; I was waiting for – for this. This is not death, dear Ralph.'

'Not for you – no. There's nothing makes us feel so much alive as to see others die. That's the sensation of life – the sense that we remain. I've had it – even I. But now I'm of no use but to give it to others. With me it's all over.' And then he paused. Isabel bowed her head further, till it rested on the two hands that were clasped upon his own. She couldn't see him now; but his far-away voice was close to her ear. 'Isabel,' he went on suddenly, 'I wish it were over for you.' [James, 2003 reprint: p. 260].

A few mornings later, Ralph is dead. Isabel tries to comfort Ralph's mother, a cold and patrician lady, but is rebuffed – again, a sudden, piercing moment, quietly stated: 'Go and thank God you've no child,' said Mrs Touchett, disengaging herself' (2003 reprint, p. 533).

To make the obvious point: even without the context of knowing precisely who these characters are, the generosity of spirit is clear, as is a kind of maturity of feeling which is missing in the case of Little Nell. Note how different the angels are in this novel compared with those that hover around the deathbed in Dickens' tale.

At times, however, there is convention alone, in the sense that we sometimes say conventional things ('I was so embarrassed I could've died'). This is from a lute song by Thomas Campion (1601), an exact contemporary of Shakespeare. He imagines his lady dead, and gone to 'shades of underground', where she can tell the story of her life:

> Then wilt thou speak of banqueting delights,
> Of masques and revels which sweet youth did make,
> Of tourneys and great challenges of knights,
> And all these triumphs for thy beauty's sake.
> When thou hast told these honours done to thee,
> Then tell, Oh, tell how thou dids't murder me.

There is little difference – except perhaps that the poetry is a bit better – between this and Tom Jones's 'It's not unusual to see me cry/I wanna die'.

Conclusion

Death in literature is a varied thing, just as is death in society. Death is also an inescapable destiny for each of us as individuals and, for this reason, has always permeated our thoughts at all levels, from the immediate sense of devastation that personal bereavement gives us to the ways in which we manage the fact of death by pushing it onto the surface, as familiarly and comfortably spooky as the deaths in Hammer horror films.

One of the uses of literature in the health professions is to help people to become more articulate about their concerns and their worries: to help them to 'talk about their feelings'. It is often said that reading literature will help health professionals themselves, perhaps particularly when they are young and lack experience; or when they are older and crusted over with the cynicism of experience. These are valuable functions, of course, but they tend to pull us away from a real sense of what literature is and can do if we study it on its own terms. The fact of the matter is that literature is difficult, and if we fail to understand it, this may be because we know too little about the cultures that have brought it into being or cannot recognise or appreciate the techniques through which it is realised, rather than because we lack the finer sentiments.

It follows from this that the role of literature as part of the growing movement in 'medical humanities' can be interpreted too narrowly. Literature, if we trust its strength and accept that to become its student is to undertake something always rich and often difficult, is a way of understanding what it is to be human. One central gift it can give to those with a scientific training is that, because it is not reductive, it can bring home the fact that there are ways of understanding that cannot be tested by multiple-choice questions. It is the role of literature to observe that the world as we experience it is irreducibly complex. An abstract of a scientific paper is one thing; an abstract of *Hamlet* is quite another, and certainly is not *Hamlet*.

References

Alcott, L. M. (1868) *Little Women*. Reprinted 1994. Penguin.

Bond, E. (1972) *Lear*. Eyre Methuen.

Campion, T. (1601) 'When thou must home to shades of underground'. Reprinted (1952) in *Elizabethan Lyrics* (ed. K. Muir). Harrap.

Diamond, J. (1999) *Because Cowards Get Cancer Too*. Vermillion.

Dickens, C. (1840–41) *The Old Curiosity Shop*. Reprinted 2001. Penguin.

Dickens, C. (1870) *The Mystery of Edwin Drood*. Reprinted (2002), ed. D. Paroissien. Penguin.

Donne, J. (*c.* 1609) 'Holy Sonnet X: Death be not proud'. Reprinted (1994) in *The Collected Poems of John Donne* (ed. R. Booth). Wordsworth Editions.

James, H. (1881) *The Portrait of a Lady*. Reprinted 2003. Penguin Classics.

Le Carré, J. (1979) *Smiley's People*. Reprinted 2000. Hodder & Stoughton.

Logue, C. (1981) *War Music*. Cape.

Moore, O. (1996) *PWA. Looking Aids in the Face*. Picador.

Nabokov, V. (1955) *Lolita*. Reprinted 1995. Penguin.

Oseko, T. (1990) *Basho's Haiku: Literal Translations for Those Who Wish to Read the Japanese Text, with Grammatical Analysis and Explanatory Notes*. Chuoh Printing.

Pope, A. (1715–20) *The Iliad of Homer*. Reprinted (1996), ed. S. Shankman. Penguin.

Pearson, H. (1946) *Oscar Wilde: His Life and Wit*. Harper Brothers.

Tennyson, A. (1849) *In memoriam A.H.H.* Reprinted (1991) as *In memoriam*, in *In Memoriam, Maud and Other Poems* (ed. J. D. Jump). Everyman.

Tyldesley, J. (1998) *Hatchepsut: The Female Pharaoh*. Penguin.

CHAPTER 8

Literary and biographical perspectives on substance use

Ed Day and Iain Smith

The effects of psychoactive drugs have been closely linked to all forms of literature for two centuries, but although alcohol has been a common theme, other drugs have not been as well represented in mainstream publishing until the past few decades. However, the escalation of the drug problem in the Western world has had an influence on popular fiction and led to a rekindling of interest in an older literature that explored these themes. The work of the 19th-century Romantics and of the Beat Generation and counterculture of the 1960s has been developed by the 'chemical generation', with ecstasy (MDMA) joining the opiates, cocaine, cannabis, lysergic acid diethylamide (LSD) and amphetamines as a backdrop to popular fiction. This chapter will explore the links between alcohol and drugs and both fictional and autobiographical writing.

Writers and alcohol

Alcohol has often been linked to the creative process and John Sutherland, a professor of English literature in London and a self-confessed 'recovering drunk', has written extensively in this area. His book *Last Drink to LA* (2001) provides some literary signposts on the path to understanding alcohol addiction and describes his own experiences at Alcoholics Anonymous (AA). Through his attendance at AA meetings, Sutherland has come to see addicts primarily as storytellers, believing that 'telling tales (most of them tall, many of them self-serving) is one of the few things that booze makes you good at' (Sutherland, 2001: p. 73).

Analysis of the lives of many famous writers reveals evidence of heavy alcohol consumption, mental illness, physical disease, family breakdown, suicide and premature death (Post, 1994). There has been much interest in the link between alcohol and writing in the USA, particularly since the realisation that five of the first seven American-born writers awarded the Nobel Prize for Literature had alcohol-related problems (Sinclair Lewis, Eugene O'Neill, William Faulkner, Ernest Hemingway and John Steinbeck). However, it is the case of F. Scott Fitzgerald, one name omitted from this list

89

(Box 8.1), that illustrates some of the possible reasons for the link between writing and drinking alcohol – a source of speculation for academics and psychiatrists alike (Goodwin, 1988; Dardis, 1989).

There is a belief that creative people have a significant flaw in their character and that this is an integral part of their creativity. Baudelaire believed that intoxication was essential to creativity (Bold, 1982: p. 87) and Nietzsche agreed, stating that 'for art to exist, for any sort of aesthetic society or perception to exist, a certain physiological precondition is indispensable: intoxication' (Marks, 2001: p. 506). In the early 1920s, Fitzgerald often introduced himself to people at parties as an alcoholic, a

---

Box 8.1 The case of F. Scott Fitzgerald

F. Scott Fitzgerald was both a creator and chronicler of the 'Roaring Twenties' in America and he achieved fame and fortune at a young age for his unique writing style. Born in 1896, by the age of 24 he was selling stories to a national newspaper for $2500 each, and his ability to turn out high-quality pieces enabled him to earn the money to maintain a lavish lifestyle of parties and drinking. Early in his career Fitzgerald tried to keep drinking and writing separate and he abstained from alcohol while writing his most famous novel *The Great Gatsby* (1925). However, by the late 1920s, he was beginning to feel the pressure of producing a follow-up to *Gatsby* and rounds of all-night parties repeatedly forced him to abandon plans for writing a new novel in favour of producing short stories for cash.

From 1928 he was beginning to use alcohol to assist his writing, regarding it as a stimulant that would fuel his creative powers. However, it seems that he was aware of the problems that it caused him, writing that 'a short story can be written on the bottle, but for a novel you need the mental speed that enables you to keep the whole pattern in your head' (Dardis, 1989: p. 123).

In 1931 he moved to Hollywood to work as a scriptwriter and, although this earned good money, he was ultimately sacked for drunken behaviour at a party. He began to find it difficult to sell his stories and 1933 saw his first alcohol-related admission to hospital. Still he continued to drink and when his next novel *Tender is The Night* was finally published in 1934, it fell below the standards expected of him. Critics agreed that the man who began the book in 1925 was not the same man that finished it in 1933 and Fitzgerald himself believed that alcohol had marred the work (Dardis, 1989).

In 1936, he wrote three short articles for a magazine that described his emotional collapse (which were ultimately published under the title *The Crack-Up* in 1945), but he avoided any mention of alcohol. The following year he took an overdose but managed to return to another job in Hollywood, which gave him the inspiration for his final (unfinished) novel *The Last Tycoon* (1941).

In the last decade of his life, Fitzgerald experienced worsening physical problems related to alcohol and underwent frequent hospital admissions; insomnia and morning drinking became regular and disabling parts of life. He finally died of a myocardial infarction in 1940, aged just 44 (Dardis, 1989).

tactic apparently designed to shock. Many writers comment on their use of alcohol to help them to relax after an intense period of work. Ernest Hemingway, a close friend of Fitzgerald, would get up early each day, write in the morning, fish or hunt in the afternoon and drink to relax and unwind in the evening. Both he and William Faulkner said that they used alcohol to help them stop writing: to switch off the creative process.

Alcohol may give writers confidence and help them to overcome what Georges Simenon called 'stage fright': the doubts about their ability to write and the quality of their work (Goodwin, 1988: p. 186). Some writers have asserted that alcohol improved their writing ability, and Fitzgerald felt that stories he wrote while sober seemed 'stupid' and 'all reasoned out, not felt'. However, sustained use of alcohol appears to have accelerated a decline in Fitzgerald's standard of both writing and health, and an opposing point of view was voiced by Stephen King when he said that 'a writer who drinks carefully is probably a better writer' (Goodwin, 1988: p. 187).

From a medical perspective, it is easy to view the life of Fitzgerald and others as being destroyed by alcohol. However, as Beveridge & Yorston (1999) point out, writers and artists have often seen the role of alcohol very differently. Alcohol has formed part of religious practices and customs for thousands of years and may be seen as an agent of mystical transport (Edwards, 2000). Writers such as Malcolm Lowry and Jack Kerouac have cited it as a means of spiritual exploration and a way of seeking enlightenment. Furthermore, drinking has often formed an integral part of literary 'scenes', where it has acted as a symbol of rebellion against contemporary values. Some authors have needed to experience degradation to produce great work. A striking example of this was the poet and author Charles Bukowski, who wrote a string of semi-autobiographical novels about his impoverished early life and his time spent drinking heavily in seedy bars. His ultimate elevation to being rich and famous appears to have vindicated his life of excessive drinking and bad behaviour (Sounes, 1998).

Donald Goodwin (1988) believes in the idea that writers are introverted and lonely people, tortured souls that can express their overload of feelings only through writing. Artists have often been portrayed as people who are especially aware of the suffering of the world and need to numb themselves to cope. Such a perspective allows an unlimited licence for hedonistic excess, leading to a long list of writers who died prematurely (including Dylan Thomas, Brendan Behan, Jack Kerouac, Malcolm Lowry and Fitzgerald himself).

However, the final piece in the jigsaw may come from a study conducted by Nancy Andreasen (1987). She rated a group of writers attending a creative writing workshop and a control group of non-writers (matched for age, gender, education and IQ) using the Research Diagnostic Criteria (RDC). The writers had significantly higher levels of bipolar disorder and alcoholism than the control group, 24 out of 30 having experienced an affective disorder at some point in their life.

Felix Post's work has also concluded that, compared with people showing other kinds of creative achievement, creative writers are excessively prone to depressive and perhaps to manic disorders, as well as to alcoholism (Post, 1994). In a study focusing on those writing poetry, fiction and plays, Post found evidence of psychopathology in the biographies of 93 out of 100 individuals (Post, 1996). These studies point to an association between creative verbal ability and affective psychopathology, and this might be the underlying basis that links creativity and alcohol dependence.

Addiction and the art of writing

The visual, auditory, emotional and cognitive effects of taking psychoactive drugs combine to form a very subjective experience, which is further influenced by the setting in which substance use occurs. Although the drug may lead an individual to new perspectives on life, describing these to others may not have the same profound effect, and therefore the deep meaning attributed to some drug experiences is seldom conveyed in a convincing manner. Nevertheless, there is a strong historical link between psychoactive substances and creativity. From the Romantic poets of the 18th century to the Beat Generation of the mid-20th, drugs have long been reputed to be central to the literary process. Even now the idea persists in print that mind-altering drugs may be a means of self-exploration and self-actualisation, and an aid to the imagination (Vayne, 2006).

Several examples have been given of the direct role that opium played in the creation of literary works of the 18th and 19th centuries (Hayter, 1968). At this time, the drug was widely available throughout Europe and a variety of preparations could be bought over the counter. Laudanum, a drink consisting of opium mixed with alcohol, was particularly popular and many people used it as an effective means of pain relief. Opium carried with it a seductive air of Far Eastern mystique and its 'specific power' to enhance dreams and memories appealed to many writers (Plant, 1999).

One example of opium-induced creativity is 'Kubla Khan, or a Vision in a Dream', a poem written by Samuel Taylor Coleridge in the late 1790s and first published in 1816. Coleridge called the poem 'a psychological curiosity' (Plant, 1999: p. 10) and claimed that it was a fragment of a much longer sequence that came to him in a dream induced by a dose of opium. Originally, the poem consisted of 200–300 lines, but when he woke up and began to write it down 'a person on business from Porlock' (Plant, 1999: p. 10) interrupted him. This was enough to break his flow and on returning to the poem he was left with only eight or ten lines and images. The fact that he later tried to recreate the situation without success did not deter others from experimenting with the drug. In Sadie Plant's words, 'poets were enchanted by the possibility that such poetry could spring from the opiated edge of waking life' (Plant, 1999: p. 11). Mary Shelley's *Frankenstein, Or the Modern Prometheus* (1818) is another well-known story to have emerged in a similar way and *The Bride of Lammermoor* (1819) by Sir Walter Scott is also reputed to have been dictated while he was taking large doses of laudanum for severe stomach pain.

Wilkie Collins was one of the most popular authors of the mid- to late-19th century. For many years, he suffered from painful physical complaints, including gout and pains in the eyes, and had used laudanum regularly for at least 20 years before he wrote his novel *The Moonstone* (1868). He is reported to have dictated the last part of the book largely under the influence of opium, and when it was finished he was not only 'pleased and astonished' at the finale, but 'did not recognise it as his own' (Hayter, 1968: p. 259). The book is about the theft of a large diamond (the Moonstone) by a man under the influence of opium who is left with no memory of his actions. Only when the scene is recreated does he find himself remembering what he has done. Opium clearly played a significant part in the author's life and it also appears in some of his other novels, including *The Woman in White* (1860), *No Name* (1862) and *Armadale* (1866).

However, perhaps the best-known writer of the time using opiates was Thomas De Quincey, who wrote extensively about the use of the drug in his book *Confessions of an English Opium Eater* (1822). Here he described the magical effects that opium had on him, allowing him to slow things down and to enhance his dreams with his own fantasies. He described a 'Dark Interpreter', a figure that allowed him to keep track of the thoughts that were arranging and rearranging themselves in his head. At first he was delighted by opium's effects, but his deficit of dreams before using it became a surfeit and he found it difficult to cope with them. Their sheer volume and complexity became almost unbearable and his mind was invaded by 'flash-back anticipations, sudden recollections and unpredicted twists' (Plant, 1999: p. 14). Although his descriptions of his dreams of oriental travel enthralled his readers when they were published, to him they became terrible nightmares. He lost the ability to distinguish between an increasingly hallucinatory waking life and the intensity of opiated dreams. He felt that his audience failed to understand the sheer intensity of these dreams, the terrifying worlds onto which his doors of perception could open.

It is not just the opiate class of drugs that has exerted a powerful influence over writers and their storytelling: hashish (also known as marijuana or cannabis depending on context and the exact preparation) has had a prominent role over many centuries. Thirteenth-century Sufi literature contains poems praising hashish for its 'meanings' and 'significances', and the state of illumination that it can produce (Boon, 2002: p. 127). Numerous folk tales from the Middle East and Muslim Central Asia make reference to hashish, as do the stories that make up the *One Thousand and One Nights* collection. In his *Travels*, published in several languages in the late 13th century, Marco Polo reported the legend of Hasan-i Sabbah or Aloadin, the Old Man of the Mountain, a medieval warlord said to have tricked young men into fighting for him by drugging them and bringing them to a paradise-like garden. The legend of Aloadin was told and retold in different forms for centuries, with hashish increasingly identified (probably incorrectly) as the offending 'drug'. Strong echoes of the legend are found in the work of Charles Baudelaire and his experiments with drug-induced 'artificial paradises' (Rudgley, 2001: p. 105). Baudelaire was a member of the Club des Hashishins, a group of artists and writers who met to share hashish-inspired 'dreams' in Paris between 1845 and 1849. Their experiences, along with those of other users of cannabis, contrast with the opium visions of the English Romantics described above in both imagery and subjectivity. As Boon comments, 'hashish can only exaggerate or develop what is already there in consciousness, it cannot "give visions"' (Boon, 2002: p. 136).

Contemporary examples of the influence of psychoactive substances on writing include *On the Road* (1957) by Jack Kerouac, which was apparently written in a 3-week burst of stimulant-fuelled creativity, and William S. Burroughs' *The Naked Lunch* (1959). Will Self's highly original and unusual work has been linked to his much-publicised problems with alcohol and drugs. However, further reflections on such legends of drug-fuelled writing often reveal them to be at least partly enhanced by fiction. Rather like the problems that Fitzgerald, Hemingway and others found in using alcohol, in reality very little good work appears to have been produced under the direct influence of drugs. Careful analysis of the manuscripts of both *The Moonstone* and *The Bride of Lammermoor* suggests that they were largely completed before or after the authors' periods of illness (Sutherland, 1998). There is also evidence from letters written by the authors that both Kerouac and Burroughs preferred to write the bulk of their work while free from drugs, and the now-abstinent Will Self comments that he has 'always had to fight against them in order to get any serious literary work done' (Barber, 2000).

The narratives of addiction

Recent qualitative research has tried to make sense of addicts' subjective experience of their own life history in relation to their problem. One such example was based on the real-life stories of 51 individuals who had overcome some form of addiction, with the researchers identifying five types of story (Hanninen & Koski-Jannes, 1999).

- *The 'AA' story* This is the least surprising, given the worldwide influence of Alcoholics Anonymous (AA) and the extension of the organisation's explanatory model to many types of problematic behaviour. The trajectory of addiction is towards destruction, with individuals beginning to gain insight only when they reach their own 'personal gutter'. At this point, they can find salvation through applying the principles of AA, a process involving humility, finding the support of fellow recovering addicts and making amends where possible. Moral absolution and self-forgiveness follow from this disease model of addiction.

- *The 'personal growth' story* Here the addict's wishes and emotions were disregarded by people around them in childhood and the addiction has arisen as a denial of the their own emotional needs in favour of those of others. Recovery results from recognising and following these true emotions through self-discovery.

- *The 'co-dependence' story* The narrative is one where repressed secrets from childhood underlie the self-abusive behaviour of addiction, and the cure relies on becoming aware of and facing up to these memories.

- *The 'love' story* Addictive behaviour compensates for a lack of love in childhood and a cure comes through finding love.

- *The 'mastery' story* This was most commonly found in relation to addiction to tobacco. It was portrayed as a battle for autonomy during the different phases of the addiction, with 'giving-up' seen as part of achieving maturity.

Work by Biernacki (1986) and Granfield & Cloud (2001) has suggested that an important part of the process of recovery from substance dependence is the ability to create or re-create an identity as a non-addict. When narratives of recovery from substance dependence are analysed, they can be seen to form an important part in constructing this sense of self. McIntosh & McKeganey (2000) describe three key areas where the narratives can be seen to be doing the work of reconstructing a non-addict identity:

- re-interpretation of the addict lifestyle – examples include the realisation that drugs gradually cease to be pleasurable but instead become necessary just to 'feel normal', or comparing the artificial confidence achieved by using drugs with the true confidence associated with being drug-free;

- reconstructing the sense of self – the sense of self while using drugs is often contrasted with the sort of person the individual believes they were before they started using drugs;

- providing explanations for recovery – being able to provide a convincing explanation for recovery can be an important part of forming of a non-addict identity. A strong reason for quitting can add extra authority to claims of having recovered, and helps to rebut the frequent challenges to this recovery. Reaching rock-bottom is often given as such a reason, and has strong parallels with the AA story mentioned above.

McIntosh & McKeganey point out that addiction narratives are often influenced by cultural factors and interactions with people around the narrator. Interaction with treatment professionals often leads to a reworking of a narrative, and there is a clear parallel between addicts' own accounts of their recovery and the characterisations of the recovery process found in the addictions literature.

The confessional narrative in the form of autobiography or memoir has increased in popularity in the latter half of the 20th century, and the addict's story fits well into the popular psychology genre. Whereas heavy use of alcohol and drugs had previously been seen as morally wrong, addiction has also become less stigmatised, leading to a broadening of the topic. It is now not uncommon to see narrative accounts of the struggle with behavioural addictions, including gambling, food and sex (Hurwitz et al, 2007).

Humans tell stories to make sense of their lives, and use this process to cope with suffering. Arthur Frank's book *The Wounded Storyteller: Body, Illness, and Ethics* (1995) highlights the value of illness narratives, the stories people tell about their experience of illness. When a person becomes ill they can lose the map that had previously guided their life, forcing them to begin to think differently. This process is achieved by experiencing their story being shared. Frank describes three types of illness narrative. The 'restitution' narrative arises most naturally to describe an acute illness, and consists of a description of being ill, recovering and returning to a pre-illness state of health. The illness is seen as transitory, with the body returning to its former image of itself before illness. The 'chaos' narrative can result when the restitution narrative breaks down, and in many ways is the opposite of restitution as its plot imagines life never getting better. Finally the 'quest' narrative does not try to avoid or downplay illness, but rather accepts it and seeks to use it. Like the story of a mythical hero, the quest narrative has a 'departure', a period of 'initiation' (where the hero is tested) and a 'return' (with the hero either boastful or humbled by his achievements). Rather than telling others what they should do in order to return to their former state, quest narratives describe the experience and share wisdom gained from it.

Although the 20th century increasingly saw addiction cast as a medical disorder requiring treatment, most addiction narratives go beyond a simple restitution form. The influence of the Alcoholics Anonymous Fellowship has led to an inherently spiritual component to many stories, particularly if they are told from the perspective of recovery. A key component of the AA meeting is the telling and retelling of life stories as a therapeutic tool, and the fourth, fifth, eighth and ninth steps of AA's Twelve Steps involve examining the individual's own life story. As recovery means more than simply not using the substance, but rather a striving for global health and happiness, many stories of recovery take the quest format. Examples include *Addicted* (1998) by the footballer Tony Adams, and *Drinking: A Love Story* (1996) by Caroline Knapp. In the latter, Knapp takes the reader through the phases of her alcoholism and outlines the help she found in AA. In common with other such stories she identifies a void within herself that alcohol filled, and describes the process of finding a sense of fulfilment without the need for external props. Other stories, such as Ann Marlowe's *How to Stop Time: Heroin from A to Z* (1999) and James Frey's *A Million Little Pieces* (2003) reject the Alcoholics/Narcotics Anonymous pathway, although they have a similar quest-like narrative structure. The production of Frey's account has a fascinating story in itself, which reveals much of the complexity of the addiction narrative (Box 8.2).

Box 8.2 Fact or fiction? The case of James Frey

A Million Little Pieces (2003) is an account of the author James Frey's stay in a drug rehabilitation centre. It begins with his admission to the clinic with four front teeth missing, a broken nose, a hole in his cheek and his eyes swollen shut. He is told by medical staff that he will die if he does not stop misusing alcohol, cocaine and a range of other substances. What follows is an incident-packed account of his 2-month stay and includes some memorable moments. He undergoes double root canal surgery without anaesthesia or pain killers, has fights with other residents, defies the strict centre rules about relationships with the opposite gender, rescues his girlfriend Lilly from a local crack house, and shares a variety of stories of past exploits with both therapists and other residents. He befriends a range of characters, including a renowned gangster, a judge and a former boxing world champion. Throughout his stay he repeats that he is 'an alcoholic, a drug addict and a criminal', but rejects the Twelve Step treatment philosophy of the centre, preferring to rely on his own mantra: 'Hold on'. The book contains powerful descriptions of his craving for substances and of the guilt associated with his past behaviour and its impact on family and friends. He avoids sentimentality about his problems, and emphasises throughout that he is difficult to love. It is this honesty, combined with an original and dynamic style of writing, that evokes powerful feelings in the reader and makes the account hard to put down.

On publication the book was promoted as 'a heartbreaking memoir'. It sold well initially, and when it was promoted by the Oprah Winfrey book club in late 2005 it moved to head the *New York Times* Best Seller List for paperback non-fiction. However, in January 2006 an investigative website The Smoking Gun reported that one of the key scenes in the book was not all it seemed to be. Frey describes hitting a policeman with his car while under the influence of crack cocaine, then resisting arrest, assaulting a police officer and trying to incite a riot. While in the rehabilitation centre he discovers that he will receive a 3-year prison sentence for these crimes, and the event has a great impact on the remainder of the book. However, The Smoking Gun revealed that he had actually received only two tickets for traffic violations and spent just 5 hours in custody. Other areas of Frey's account were also shown to have been embellished and many readers felt betrayed, as the book conveyed the idea of triumph over adversity in such a powerful way that it had become a source of great hope.

It emerged that Frey had offered the book as fiction to a number of publishers before reworking it as a non-fiction memoir. Many addicts in recovery had commented that the book seemed far-fetched before the news broke, but Frey still says that the bulk of his book is true, pointing out that most memoirs (as opposed to autobiography) contain truth and fiction side by side. In many ways the book symbolises the place of addiction within narrative, lying somewhere between fact and fiction. As Hurwitz *et al* (2007: p. 485) suggest, readers should be wary of taking addiction narratives at face value, as hidden in the detail 'there may be the lineaments of a revelation relating to something that has nothing to do with addiction per se but which turns out to be the major subject of the narrative'.

Despite these insights from autobiographical accounts, an important feature of addiction is often the individual's denial of their problem. Fictional accounts may help us gain a greater understanding of this issue. As one author has observed, 'an addiction is held in place by an elaborate system of deceptions' (Beard, 1996), and a good fictional example of this is Joseph Roth's 1939 novella *The Legend of the Holy Drinker*. This follows the fortunes of Andreas, an alcoholic vagrant who drinks as a response to external circumstances, and is a simple story that engenders pathos and has parallels in Roth's own life story. Alternative narratives are also provided by Burroughs' *Junky* (first published pseudonomously in 1953 under the title *Junkie: Confessions of an Unredeemed Drug Addict*) and Welsh's *Trainspotting* (1993), in which the addiction and its maintenance are seen as a matter of personal choice rather than something over which the individual has no control. This is no surprise when we consider the perspective of attribution theory outlined in the work of John Booth Davies. In *The Myth of Addiction* he suggests that 'most people who use drugs do so for their own reasons, on purpose, because they like it, and because they find no adequate reason for not doing so' (Davies, 1997: p. xi). However, the capacity to blame the properties of the drug or external circumstances for its repeated use seems to predominate in our culture and this is reflected in much of the writing cited in this review.

A further dimension brought out in literature is the polarisation between warning against the dangers of drugs and alcohol on the one hand, and arguing that drug experiences are life-enhancing on the other. In the face of this dichotomy, some of the more interesting literature, such as *Junky*, occupies a middle ground in taking a more matter-of-fact approach. The 'harder' drugs (heroin, cocaine) are mostly represented in the scare stories, whereas the psychedelic drugs (LSD, ecstasy) fall at the life-enhancement end of the spectrum. As an example, compare *Junk* (Burgess, 1996) and *Iced* (Shell, 1993) with *The Doors of Perception* (Huxley, 1954).

Doctors and addiction

How do addicted patients view their doctors? A literary insight is given by William Burroughs in *Junky*, written in the 1950s when doctors were the main source of heroin. He describes them disparagingly as 'croakers' and gives advice on how best to approach them in order to achieve the addict's goal of receiving a prescription. He prefers a convincing story that allows the doctor to save face in writing the prescription rather than a 'factual approach', and advises the reader that 'you need a good bedside manner with doctors or you will get nowhere' (Burroughs, 1997 reprint: p. 21). Although this account was written in the American context and before the current vogue for substitute prescribing, there are still lessons to be learned from it.

There are few literary accounts of doctors who successfully help patients with addiction to overcome their problems, perhaps reflecting the reality that recovery is about self-discovery. Research suggests that the impact of treatment is modest in the long term and that recovery is about the individual constructing a new identity that does not revolve around drugs or alcohol and acknowledging the need to abstain. One exception is the writer Eugene O'Neill who, after many failed attempts at recovery from his heavy alcohol use, sustained prolonged abstinence after psychoanalysis (Ludwig, 1988).

In contrast, many accounts exist of unscrupulous doctors who produce addiction in their patients. An excellent example of this is the doctor in Hubert Selby Junior's *Requiem for a Dream* (1978). Not only does the doctor lead the mother of a son addicted to street drugs into dependence on diet pills; he then tries to counteract her descent into psychosis with tranquillisers, giving little time or thought to the consequences of the prescription. Doctors who have themselves become impaired through the use of drugs and alcohol frequently appear in literature. Some commentators have suggested that drug and alcohol misuse is the single most important factor when considering the impairment of doctors' health and performance (Fowlie, 1999), and perhaps this literary concern reflects not only reality but also an interest in the complexity of character found in such individuals. Although he was unable to accept his own problem with alcohol, Fitzgerald wrote memorably about the psychiatrist Dick Diver and his descent into alcoholism in *Tender is the Night* (1934). There are also some notable short stories on this theme, including Mikhail Bulgakov's *Morphine* (1927). This is a warning against the perils of self-medicating with drugs and the addictive process that might ensue, as the doctor Polyakov ultimately takes his own life. Finally, Verghese's *The Tennis Partner: A Doctor's Story of Friendship and Loss* (1998) is a personal narrative by an American physician who becomes aware of an addictive disorder in a junior colleague who is an ex-tennis professional. The author relates the problem of addiction in the medical profession to the expectation that doctors should conceal their own emotions and to the possibility that vulnerable individuals may be left in a position of isolation.

The use of literary and narrative studies to teach about addiction

There are good grounds to use the materials we describe here as an adjunct to medical education, and the document *Tomorrow's Doctors* (General Medical Council, 1993) has already encouraged the growth of the disciplines of medical humanities and narrative-based medicine. A number of special study modules running in UK medical schools draw on these themes and thus help foster an awareness of patients' possible explanatory stories about their addiction. Such studies also help show that although addiction and drug-taking are often portrayed as a new phenomenon, this is far from the case. This area of study can also lead to challenges to orthodoxy, such as Theodore Dalrymple's *Romancing Opiates: Pharmacological Lies and the Addiction Bureaucracy* (2006). Here, writing under a pen name, the much published medical author Anthony Daniels (a retired prison doctor and psychiatrist) argues that we have bought into a concept of heroin dependence that was produced by the literary tradition described above and that this has influenced public opinion and the medical response. Such material can provoke useful debate in small-group medical teaching.

Conclusion

We hope that we have shown that a study of narrative and literature is capable of broadening our perspective on the phenomena of addiction and substance use. Modern diagnostic concepts and operational definitions of misuse and dependence tend to simplify a complex problem, and literary accounts help us to regain the perspective of the highly individual experience of using the different classes of psychoactive drugs. Furthermore we have touched on new qualitative research on addicts' own narratives of their dependence which appears to complement this literary perspective. Finally, we have warned against taking too seriously the claims of drug-enhanced creativity made by some authors and also found literary warnings of our own vulnerabilities, as doctors, to addictive disorders.

References

Andreasen, N. C. (1987) Creativity and mental illness: prevalence rates in writers and their first-degree relatives. *American Journal of Psychiatry*, **144**, 1288–1292.

Barber, L. (2000) Self control. *The Observer*, 11 June (http://books.guardian.co.uk/departments/generalfiction/story/0,6000,330140,00.html).

Beard, R. (1996) *X20*. Flamingo.

Beveridge, A. & Yorston, G. (1999) I drink, therefore I am: alcohol and creativity. *Journal of the Royal Society of Medicine*, **92**, 646–648.

Biernacki, P. (1986) *Pathways From Heroin Addiction. Recovery Without Treatment*. Temple University Press.

Bold, A. (ed.) (1982) *Drink to Me Only: The Prose (and Cons) of Drinking*. Robin Clark.

Boon, M. (2002) *The Road of Excess: A History of Writers on Drugs*. Harvard University Press.

Burroughs, W. S. (1953) *Junkie: Confessions of an Unredeemed Drug Addict*. Reprinted (1977) as *Junky*. Penguin Books.

Dalrymple, T. (2006) *Romancing Opiates: Pharmacological Lies and the Addiction Bureaucracy*. Encounter Books.

Dardis, T. (1989) *The Thirsty Muse: Alcohol and the American Writer*. Ticknor & Fields.

Davies, J. B. (1997) *The Myth of Addiction* (2nd edn). Harwood Academic Publishers.

Edwards, G. (2000) *Alcohol. The Ambiguous Molecule*. Penguin Books.

Fowlie, D. (1999) The misuse of alcohol and other drugs by doctors: a UK report and one region's response. *Alcohol and Alcoholism*, **5**, 666–671.

Frank, A. W. (1995) *The Wounded Storyteller: Body, Illness, and Ethics.* University of Chicago Press.

General Medical Council (1993) *Tomorrow's Doctors.* GMC.

Goodwin, D. W. (1988) *Alcohol and the Writer.* Andrews and McMeel.

Granfield, R. & Cloud, W. (2001) Social context and "natural recovery": the role of social capital in the resolution of drug-associated problems. *Substance Use and Misuse,* **36,** 1543–1570.

Hanninen, V. & Koski-Jannes, A. (1999) Narratives of recovery from addictive behaviour. *Addiction,* **94,** 1837–1848.

Hayter, A. (1968) *Opium and the Romantic Imagination.* Faber & Faber.

Hurwitz, B., Tapping, C. & Vickers, N. (2007) Life histories and narratives of addiction. In *Drugs and the Future: Brian Science, Addiction and Society* (eds D. Nutt, T. W. Robbins, G. V. Stimson, *et al*). Academic Press.

Ludwig, A. M. (1988) *Understanding the Alcoholic's Mind.* Oxford University Press.

Marks, H. (ed.) (2001) *The Howard Marks Book of Dope Stories.* Vintage.

McIntosh, J. & McKeganey, N. (2000) Addicts' narratives of recovery from drug use: constructing a non-addict identity. *Social Science and Medicine,* **50,** 1501–1510.

Plant, S. (1999) *Writing on Drugs.* Faber & Faber.

Post, F. (1994) Creativity and psychopathology. A study of 291 world-famous men. *British Journal of Psychiatry,* **165,** 22–34.

Post, F. (1996) Verbal creativity, depression and alcoholism. An investigation of one hundred American and British writers. *British Journal of Psychiatry,* **168,** 545–555.

Rudgley, R. (ed.) (2001) *Wildest Dreams: An Anthology of Drug-Related Literature.* Abacus.

Sounes, H. (1998) *Charles Bukowski: Locked in the Arms of a Crazy Life.* Rebel.

Sutherland, J. (1998) Turns unstoned. *Times Literary Supplement,* 30 October.

Sutherland, J. (2001) *Last Drink to LA.* Short Books.

Vayne, J. (2006) *Pharmakon: Drugs and the Imagination.* Mandrake.

CHAPTER 9

Dementia and literature

Christopher A. Vassilas

There is an increasing awareness among the general public of the terms dementia and Alzheimer's disease and of how these illnesses manifest themselves. This recognition has been reflected in the arts. Richard Eyre's film *Iris*, based on the biography of Iris Murdoch (Bayley, 1998), was released in 2001. More recently two long-running UK soap operas, *The Archers* (on BBC Radio 4) and *Coronation Street* (ITV television), have both featured characters who have developed Alzheimer's disease. Several major authors have published books exploring the experience of dementia. I have selected five of these books which give an insight into the devastating condition of dementia from differing perspectives. Two are fictional works: *Out of Mind* by J. Bernlef (1984) and *Scar Tissue* by Michael Ignatieff (1993), the latter being an observational account of a mother's decline that could be described as an autobiographical novel. Three are non-fictional accounts: John Bayley's book *Iris* has more of the elements of a conventional biography, whereas *Remind Me Who I Am, Again* by Linda Grant (1998) is both a biography of her mother and the story of a generation of Jews that fled the pogroms in Eastern Europe for a better life in the West; *Untold Stories* (Bennett, 2005), the title piece of a collection of writings published under that name by the writer Alan Bennett, is a memoir of his family and the last part details his mother's experience of dementia.

Out of Mind

J. Bernlef is the pseudonym of the Dutch novelist and poet Hendrik Jan Marsman. *Out of Mind* is the English-language translation of the 1984 novel *Hersenschimmen*, which established Marsman's reputation as a writer. *Out of Mind* is the most imaginative and difficult of the works I discuss here. Bernlef has thought himself into the mind of a 74-year-old man who appears suddenly to develop cognitive impairment and rapidly deteriorates over a seemingly short period. Whereas authors such as Grant and Ignatieff go out of their way to talk about the scientific aspects of dementia, Bernlef gives an impressionistic, first-person account. The book is interesting because, like all novels, it needs coherence in order to communicate to the reader yet it attempts to illuminate how a disintegrated mind works.

How does Bernlef approach this task? He gradually describes the breakdown of his protagonist Maarten, a Netherlander living with his wife Vera in the USA. Over one winter Maarten experiences a disintegration of his mental faculties. Initially, there are small lapses: he realises that it is afternoon when he had thought that it was morning; he lets his tea grow cold, not noticing this until his wife points it out: 'How could I have forgotten! And tea? I could have sworn it was morning' (Bernlef, 1988 reprint: p. 3). He knows that his memory is failing, but justifies it: 'I always did have a poor memory' (p. 5). However, over the first few pages of the book it becomes clear to us that Maarten does not have a full understanding of what is going on around him. One morning he finds that he cannot get out of the house; realising that the doors are locked and that he cannot find his keys, he gets a hammer and screwdriver and prises the front door open. The logicality of his actions is quite clear: he has encountered a problem and found what he believes is the best solution for it. He goes for a walk with his dog and believes that he must attend a meeting in a certain house; the house that he approaches is empty so he breaks in. When he then realises that he should not be in the house and that he has done something wrong by breaking in Bernlef captures his consternation: 'What am I doing here? In the summer, people from Boston live here ... I may get into trouble over this' (p. 36).

There is an inexorable decline as the illness progresses. People he sees in town become mixed up in his mind with people he knew many years ago. Deeper into the book, Vera, on the advice of a doctor, takes out a photograph album to show Maarten. The photographs trigger memories of the past, of the Second World War and life in occupied Holland, which Maarten shares with his wife. However, this is just a temporary respite, and he begins to believe that he is in his childhood home back in Europe. Later, a carer again produces a photograph album, but as Maarten's illness has progressed he can hardly recognise any of the figures. The carer presses and asks him whether he recognises a woman in a photograph (it is Vera): ' "Mama I suppose. My mother, I mean, I beg your pardon. With me." I look from the photograph to her face. "Or am I wrong?" ' (p. 101). Memories of life in Holland during the war are released and Maarten talks about them to his carer, but it is as if he does not know where they are coming from: 'I talk and talk and it is as if I am talking myself out of history, as if this were a book from which I am reading, or a text I know by heart; one thing is clear; what you tell you lose' (p. 102).

When the doctor calls for the first time to assess Maarten we see things entirely from Maarten's viewpoint. Although he is clearly an intelligent man he simply does not know who the doctor is, despite being introduced to him, or why he is there. Throughout the book Maarten strives to discern meaning in the world. He finds it, but it is mediated through his dementia and fluctuates from minute to minute. As Maarten struggles, Vera desperately tries to cope with his illness.

The text does not give Maarten's diagnosis, but he seems to have a rapidly progressive dementia, perhaps of a vascular type with sudden onset and periods of unexpected deterioration. The narrative, like his illness, lurches from situation to situation, with events suddenly erupting. For instance, when Maarten wants to let the dog into the house he breaks a window for it to jump through. Nevertheless, even as he becomes more severely impaired he can momentarily understand what is going on, as when he overhears Vera talking about him and his illness. Elements of his life are remembered in fragments: we learn about his early loves and how he met Vera, his working life and the dislocation of moving from Europe to the USA.

Eventually Maarten is placed in an institution. At some level he is aware of people around him, describing them as 'drugged it would seem by the way they sit staring in front of them at the whitewashed wall' (p. 120). But his ability to construct meaning becomes more and more limited. The deterioration in the way the language is structured in the book parallels the fragmentation of Maarten's mind. In the early chapters there are well-constructed sentences such as 'I smile into Vera's mocking green eyes with dark flecks in the pupils. The other day I came across an old photograph of her' (p. 3). By the time Maarten is in the nursing home his sentences are broken up and barely comprehensible: 'go on drinking...rinse...rinse...rinse...stream...I must stream...stream away...why do those cards remove this body from its fountainhead and dry it and lead it away from the water?' (p. 129).

The questions raised in this book are not just about dementia. Bernlef is interested in how we all make sense of the world and in what leads to our sense of identity. At the beginning Maarten wishes 'If only spring would come soon' (p. 11); by the end of the book, as his grasp of the world fades away, he can no longer make sense of the information he is given. He hears the voice of a woman, whom we assume is Vera, telling him that winter is over and spring is about to start; but he no longer recognises her 'she says...she whispers...the spring which is about to begin...'(p. 130).

Iris: A Memoir of Iris Murdoch

In the UK, perhaps the best-known account of Alzheimer's disease is the biography of Iris Murdoch, one of the best-regarded post-war British novelists, written by her husband, the academic John Bayley. Iris is a striking story of love and illness because of the milieu in which she and John Bayley lived. They met and courted in post-war Oxford, in what now seems a completely different world. Iris Murdoch is portrayed as an exotic bohemian creature who had little regard for the sexual mores of the time. She was a bright student who studied, and later taught, philosophy at Oxford University. John Bayley was, by his own account, a socially awkward man who fell in love with her and had to adapt to her lifestyle.

Although there is sadness in the story it is also a celebration of a life and of world-class achievements. Their life together is detailed and the book is shot through with poignant examples of how Iris's past life relates to her condition at the end: 'She does not know she has written twenty-seven remarkable novels, as well as her books on philosophy; received honorary doctorates from all the major universities; become a Dame of the British Empire' (p. 41).

Throughout their marriage the couple loved to swim, particularly in fresh water, Iris often naked. The book begins by describing the two of them going for a swim, contrasting the ease and naturalness of what used to be with the difficulties of the present dealing with someone who has dementia: 'Once we would have got our clothes off as soon as possible and slid silently into the water ... Now I had quite a struggle getting Iris's clothes off ... She protested, gently though vigorously, as I levered off the outer layers' (p. 40).

John first realises that something is wrong when Iris is in Israel, taking part in a discussion at an international conference. She suddenly finds it difficult in front of the large audience to come out with the words to reply to questions, something with which she had previously been quite at ease. Although Bayley does not explicitly say that he knows what the diagnosis is at that time, he knows that this is the start of a serious problem. That moment is encapsulated dramatically in a prestigious literary setting. Many carers of people with Alzheimer's similarly recall such moments, perhaps in more mundane settings. Often it is only in retrospect that they realise that changes have been building up over time. For John Bayley, this moment triggers the realisation that some odd remarks Iris had made a few months before about a character in one of her books had a significance he had not understood at the time. The comments were in fact a clue that she was developing Alzheimer's disease.

As the illness progresses, offers of help from friends and from professionals come in. For Bayley these are an intrusion into a very private relationship. For example, he writes 'let us postpone it while we can' and 'I'm never absent so that carers are not now needed' (p. 237). What is striking, and what we may sometimes forget, is the continuing pleasure that John and Iris take in their relationship. An unusual example of this is their routine of watching the *Teletubbies*, a television programme aimed at young children. Every morning, John would switch on the television set and this eccentric old-fashioned couple, who had never really been television watchers, would take delight together in a strange children's world.

As the illness progresses he is able to share less and less with Iris. *Teletubbies* no longer interests her and he is unable to gain any insight into what she is thinking. As he realises that he is finding it increasingly difficult to care for Iris, inevitably guilt emerges – he senses a reproachful look in Iris's face when he leaves her for an hour with a friend. The frustration and anger of dealing with someone with Alzheimer's disease gradually come to the fore. With the honesty that characterises Bayley's telling of their early courtship he chronicles his despair and anger, which are paralleled by his sense of isolation as the identity of the person he has shared his life with diminishes. He documents his rage, which spills over at Iris's continual over-watering of some house plants of which he is fond.

The book ends with a description of the events of Christmas Day 1997. By this time Iris has become totally dependent on John. They have been invited to his brother's house in London, and there is an elegiac account of their walk around the city, the comfort of a familiar ritual. Illusion sustains John and the book ends not on a note of despair, nor in unjustified optimism, but with a dignified acceptance of the illness.

Remind Me Who I Am, Again

This is Linda Grant's story of her mother Rose and how she developed dementia. Like the other books here, it is much more than a factual account of an illness. Linda Grant's grandparents were Jewish refugees who fled Eastern Europe for the USA, but were tricked and ended up in England. The book is the account not only of how Linda and her sister Michelle coped with their mother, but also of how they came to terms with their cultural heritage. Rose Grant had multi-infarct dementia and, as befits a book by a journalist on *The Guardian* newspaper, there is a good factual account of the illness and its symptoms.

The origin of this book was an article that Grant wrote for *The Guardian* of her battles with the bureaucracy of social services and that grew into a history of her family. Linda struggled to keep her mother's memories alive: 'I don't know if it's a tragedy or a blessing when Jews, who insist on forgiving and forgetting nothing, should end their lives remembering nothing' (Grant, 1998: p. 15), she says of her mother. As her mother's short-term memory fades, memories of her childhood start to come flooding back. Ironically, these are the very recollections that Linda dismissed as boring family tales when she was a child growing up in the Liverpool of 1960s' Beatlemania.

For Linda Grant the point of realisation that there is something abnormal going on occurs when she is sitting in her mother's flat in Bournemouth and Rose is repeating over and over that she wants Linda to have some sundae spoons. The difficulties the daughters have in their relationship with their mother cloud their recognition of the development of the illness and this in turn feeds into their guilt. On one occasion while staying with Michelle and her boyfriend, Rose has tantrums and runs out of the house, ending up in a cheap hotel. Only gradually do Linda and Michelle realise that the increasing arguments that their mother is having with them represent something more sinister than selfishness. In 1990, Linda takes her mother for a holiday in Sorrento: 'The week in Italy was the last time that life was, for her, what it was supposed to be' (p. 121).

The book is a chronological account and in it we can see a disease take shape and Grants' painful process of understanding what is happening to her mother: 'The problem, and it will take … a little time to work this out, is that it is not about who our mother is but who we want her to be' (p. 199).

Following a trip to Harley Street to see a specialist, Rose is diagnosed with dementia. The diagnosis itself is a relief to the two sisters, as they have a name onto which to hang the problems that their mother has been experiencing. For example, the specialist tells them that 'the long held grudges about grandchildren or bad daughters had nothing to do with anything' (p. 131.) At that point Linda and Michelle 'take on the might of the system' (p. 138) and experience a depressingly complete lack of coordination between health and social services.

There is some discussion of the moral issues involved in forcing elderly people into long-term care and Grant makes the point that by letting her mother remain at home, her 'mother's rights are allowing her to spend twenty-three hours alone, over-dosed or under-medicated, and crying' (p. 159).

Whether one believes this to be the case or not (and Rose's situation was by no means as bad as that in which many patients with dementia who are alone find themselves), the anguish and powerlessness felt by carers is impressively described.

Because Rose is Jewish the process of finding a residential home is made simpler because of an organisation called Jewish Care. However, Linda Grant finds herself up against the rules of social services funding and, as with many carers, there is a sense of incomprehension about the rules that govern whether an individual can go into residential care.

Once her mother is finally placed in a home, Linda visits her far more often than she would have done before. It is only when someone at the home points this out to her and questions who is benefiting from the visits that she is able to begin letting go. Linda Grant's accounts of the conversations she has with staff at the home show that these individuals played a major part in helping the sisters to come to terms with the situation. They read like descriptions of psychotherapy sessions. Grant realises that she does love her mother, but not like those who say 'I love my mother. I could never put her in a home. For loves are like people, each is different' (p. 286).

The issue of Jewishness and how Rose's illness made Linda face this, is a major theme of the book. Grant writes: 'All communities are to do with memory and none more so than the Jewish community in which everything is about what was' (p. 269).

Scar Tissue

The Canadian writer Michael Ignatieff's account of his mother's decline into dementia comes from a different perspective. In describing *Scar Tissue*, Ignatieff writes '[although it] was based on personal experience, the experience wasn't mine. It was my brother's. He was there. I was the absent brother' (quoted in Durrant, 2000). This is a powerful novel, in which the mother's illness triggers a crisis in the personal life of the narrator. It is a passionately told story, with elements of both philosophy and popular science. The reason given for telling this story is that it is a way of redeeming the painful memory of his mother's death by going 'back to the unscarred beginnings ... That is how she should be remembered' (p. 1). As the story develops, intimations of what is about to happen begin to intrude. The mother suddenly abandons painting – her main interest in life – with no explanation, and the narrator immediately blames his father. But in the telling of the story he begins to understand how his parents love each other and to question the anger that he has directed at his father. Imperceptibly his mother changes – instead of waiting for family meals to finish she begins to clear the table while people are still eating. There is an accumulation of incidents – first she loses her glasses, then her shoes; next, pots are left boiling on the stove. The narrator believes that his mother must have some insight and that she must at some point have understood what was happening to her.

As one would expect from an intellectual such as Ignatieff, the book is full of philosophical musings. At one point the narrator becomes fascinated by the idea that a positive mental attitude could help his mother to get better, as propounded in numerous best-selling books: 'I longed to believe that my mother was holding back the force of the illness with the power of her will' (p. 63). But he realises that this is not true, and concludes that a stoical attitude to the inevitability of death, rather than pretence that it can be cheated, is the only appropriate response.

The two brothers in the novel represent the polarisation that the narrator sees in his parents' marriage. On the one hand there is the doctor brother who, like his father, is a scientist, and on the other the narrator, a philosophy lecturer who, like his mother, has a background in the arts. The narrator believes that his father thought of him as having a 'scatty female mind, interested in gossip and personal details and stories' (p. 25). The tension between the narrator and his father permeates the book. This polarity of world views is evident when the mother is taken to hospital to see a neurologist, who is described as seeing 'a disease of memory function, with a stable name and a clear prognosis' (p. 60). For the narrator, it is different: 'I see an illness of selfhood, without a name or even a clear cause' (p. 60).

After the death of their father the two sons have to put their mother in a nursing home, the narrator's brother coming down from Boston so they can 'share out the guilt' (p. 98). Even when their mother is in the home there are still moments of happiness, albeit brief. On one occasion, the brothers take her on a car trip. During the journey they start to sing a song from their childhood; they cannot remember a rhyme, but their mother is able to complete it. The narrator is suddenly drawn to the past, to a time when the whole family were helpless with laughter, singing the same song together. The narrator's brother is fascinated in a clinical way by her response, and yet he confides, 'I'm a fifty year-old man and the thing that matters most to me, the thing that actually makes me believe I exist is the fact that an old woman who lives in a nursing home recognises me' (p. 127).

The narrator's brother has a research interest in dementia and takes him to his laboratory, where he shows him, through an electron microscope, a section of brain affected by Alzheimer's disease. There the narrator sees the characteristic neurofibrillary tangles and amyloid deposits, the scar tissue of the book's title.

At the end of the book, on learning that he has cancer, the narrator asks: 'Does understanding anything make a difference, if there is nothing you can do to stop it happening? An excellent question and one an entire life of introspection does not enable me to answer' (p. 197).

Untold Stories

In this collection of prose, Alan Bennett uses the story of his mother's mental illness in his recounting of a history of his family, the 'untold story' of the title. In this short piece, barely 12 pages long, Bennett's description of his mother's final dementia distils a huge amount of both information and reflection about the illness, picking up many of the themes of the other authors and succinctly summarising them. This is the work of a master craftsman. He writes with great humour – I laughed out loud on several occasions, even on re-reading his words – and yet at times with incredible tenderness: 'Twenty years ago she would have been as embarrassed by this affectation of affection as I am. But that person is dead, or forgotten anyway, living only in the memory of this morose middle-aged man' (p. 118).

There is a quiet honesty in the story of his mother's final days. He recounts how she had suffered from a severe recurrent depressive illness for many years, with frequent hospital admissions and electroconvulsive therapy. As she grew older that illness merged into dementia. The style of the narrative has an easy familiarity and anyone who has heard Alan Bennett speak will hear that voice when reading his prose: it disguises an unblinking frankness with which he describes both the world around him and his reactions to it.

After his father died in 1974, Bennet and his brother arranged for their mother to go into a nursing home. In a passage remembering how long ago those times seem he describes how 'when in due course blacks take their place among the patients here and in similar establishments it will, I suppose, signal a sort of victory, though hardly one to be rejoiced over as the price of it is a common enslavement to age and infirmity' (p. 113). With this he conveys a sense of the inevitability of senility, a fate awaiting all who live in contemporary Britain and take their place in society here – the democracy of senility.

There is resignation about his mother's condition and the need for her to go into a nursing home. He notes of the residents: 'They are not dying; they are just incapable of living, though capable of being long-lived nevertheless. My mother lives like this for fifteen years' (p. 117).

He acutely observes the loss of identity his mother undergoes and how the institution in which she is placed reinforces this, absorbing her into the world of the institution and away from her old life:

> [I]t isn't only the cardigan and the frock that aren't hers. She has even acquired someone else's name ... The nurses ... aren't over-particular about names and call her Lily [p. 111].
>
> 'Her name's actually Lilian,' I say primly.
> 'I know but we call her Lily' [p. 119].

Common themes

Although the books I have discussed are written from a variety of points of view, certain recurrent themes occur.

Loss of identity

Dementia is described frequently as a disease of memory, and the nature and character of memory is a preoccupation in these writings. It is an illness that destroys the person and ultimately confirms the centrality of memory to human life.

As Linda Grant puts it, 'Memory, I have come to understand, is everything, it's life itself' (1998: p. 17). This theme is echoed by all the authors. Ignatieff muses on the case of Willem de Kooning, the famous American painter who developed Alzheimer's disease and yet continued to paint: 'a painting might still be painted where there is not self to do the painting' (1993: p. 149). He uses this as an illustrative example not only to discuss where artistic creativity comes from: 'Where does art come from? From the intentional self or the primal self' (p. 153) but also to reflect on what has happened to the narrator's mother and to speculate more widely on the nature of what makes up someone's personality. In *Out of Mind* (Bernlef, 1984), the disintegration of Maarten's personality is mirrored in the prose reflecting his thoughts, the last few pages of the book being barely coherent.

Back to childhood

For observers it seems that people with dementia are regressing to their childhood: 'Second childhood in my mother's case is not just a phrase but a proper description of how skills learned in the first years of her life are gradually unlearned at its end and in reverse order: speech has come out of babble and reverts to it' (Bennett, 2005: p. 114). John Bayley describes Iris Murdoch happily watching children's programmes on the television. Of course, for the offspring of people with dementia this implies a reversal of roles: 'Now we both knew we had to become parents', Ignatieff (1993: p. 96) writes of himself and his brother, who have to look after their mother. Linda Grant puts it more succinctly: 'My mother, my child' (1998: p. 166).

Nursing homes

All of these accounts finish with admission to a nursing home, although many people with dementia are able to remain in their own homes. The horror of the family in placing a parent in a home for people with senile dementia is striking. Linda Grant's sister's initial response is 'they've chosen the wrong place, she can't possibly stay here' (1998: p. 196). As she says, 'it is not the staff who are a problem – it is the other residents' (p. 199). Iris Murdoch's mother had had Alzheimer's disease and ended up in a nursing home, so John Bayley knew through personal experience the course of the illness. He was determined to avoid Iris's move to a home for as long as possible. Nursing homes for dementia are almost invariably described as bleak, impersonal places, reflecting the illness itself. For Alan Bennett a nursing home is 'a home that is not a home', where the residents are 'not dying; they are just incapable of living' (2005: p. 117).

For many writers, admission to a home is seen as the final stage in the individual's life, their personality left behind. Associated with the decision to consign someone to a home there follows, inevitably, guilt on the part of the family. Linda Grant describes 'the frightful and guilt-inducing decision that one is to remove one's mother from all that she holds most dear and familiar' (1998: p. 173). The guilt of placing a parent in long-term care is also inescapable for the narrator in *Scar Tissue*. The last thing his mother says to him after he and his brother take her to the nursing home is 'Get out' (Ignatieff, 1993: p. 99). His next visit – he times it – lasts 7 minutes.

This guilt remains even after the loved one has moved into a home. As Linda Grant writes: 'I observed that there was a gold standard of attendance by relatives ... which I fell far short of' (1998: p. 298).

Family stories

Family stories provide an opportunity to reassess the past. For those who are children there is an attempt to make sense of how they got to where they are. Alan Bennett's account of his parents and their marriage is underlined by a fierce pride in what they achieved given the constraints of the world in which they lived. Similarly, Linda Grant says of her mother 'in her brain resided the very last links with her generation' (1998: p. 31) and her story of her parents is the story not just of one family but of a whole people who migrated from Eastern Europe. Even in Michael Ignatieff's account, as the mother's dementia progresses the narrator develops a grudging respect for the father from whom he had become estranged.

The medical profession

Doctors need to have a certain amount of detachment in order to deal daily with illness. Clinicians see patients and their carers at times of crisis, whereas literature highlights the continuity of people's lives. In dementia, the role of doctors is often seen as peripheral in an illness for which medical intervention is limited. In the accounts discussed here, interactions with doctors show them in both a favourable and an unfavourable light. Bayley writes that Iris Murdoch's diagnosis is confirmed and she is referred to hospitals by 'our own friendly harassed GP' (1998: p. 234). Linda Grant describes her mother's GP as being dismissive of her memory problems: '"Old people forget things," he says, "my own mother forgets things"' (1998: p. 123).

Doctors, of course, play a minor role in these accounts; dementia is a chronic illness cruelly lasting for many years. So what do such books offer clinicians? All doctors work within society and need to understand how the population at large see the illnesses they work with. Although the authors I have discussed have all offered a very personal and particular perspective on dementia, they also reflect how the wider world views this condition. Most old age psychiatrists will not be surprised by the content of these narratives: they are familiar from our day-to-day working. What they do reveal, however, are perspectives on dementia completely different from our own. Reminding ourselves of this will surely help us to be better doctors.

Moral issues

Writing about a person who has dementia and who may not be able to understand or reply to what is being said about them is a complex moral issue. If it is considered acceptable to publish an account of someone's dementia (whether alive or dead), then the debate turns to the degree to which the illness is described. Both *Remind Me Who I Am, Again* and *Iris* were published while the subjects were still alive (although unable to understand what had been written). There were accusations that Bayley's account of his wife's illness was unjustifiably intrusive. The most notable of these was made by A. N. Wilson, who published his own biography of Iris Murdoch (Wilson, 2003). In it, Wilson declared himself 'sickened' by Bayley's frankness about the 'intensely private' Iris and accused him of being a 'screaming hate-filled child'. Unfortunately, this debate degenerated into a feud that has been documented in the literary pages of British newspapers (Taylor, 2003).

There is no doubt that Bayley's account of his wife's dementia and the portrayal of her towards the end of her illness are sometimes uncomfortable for the reader, and there is a sense of prying uninvited into her life. From the point of view of the wider debate regarding dementia, however, John Bayley's account, whatever his motivation for writing it, has helped to encourage a more honest discussion of the effect of this crippling illness on sufferers and those who care for them. Linda Grant also airs this issue, quoting her sister on the moral dilemma of whether to 'subject your family to forensic scrutiny' (1998: p. 306); but she concludes that 'to examine life is a difficult choice … but the only meaningful one' (p. 307), echoing Socrates' statement that an unexamined life is not worth living.

Conclusion

It is a long time since Alois Alzheimer published his famous account of a patient with what came to be called Alzheimer's disease (Alzheimer, 1907), which is now recognised as the most common cause of dementia. The second most common type is vascular dementia (mostly multi-infarct dementia), although it was not until three-quarters of a century after Alzheimer's work that multi-infarct dementia was identified and properly described (Hachinski et al, 1974).

As we have learnt more about the dementias and their prevalence has increased because of the aging population, people have become more willing to talk about them. But stigma is still attached to these illnesses, and dementia today is perhaps where cancer was several decades ago: even to use the word cancer was regarded by many as taboo (Harpham & Hoel, 1997). An increasing amount of literature is being published in which dementia and its consequences are discussed, and a good list of novels, plays, poetry and short stories (albeit with a North American bias) can be found on the Alzheimer's Association website (http://www.alz.org).

Linda Grant explains why she chose to write about her mother's illness: 'Because there is a silence, a taboo. No one knows how to feel, or what to think because the meteor of dementia that strikes families and wipes out so much is supposed to be part of the realm of privacy' (1998: p. 300).

The books discussed here have collectively helped the process of breaking the taboo.

References

Alzheimer, A. (1907) Uber eine eigneartige Ehrankung der Himrinde. *Allgemeine Zeitschrift für Psychiatrie*, **64**, 146–148.

Bayley, J. (1998) *Iris: A Memoir of Iris Murdoch*. Abacus.

Bennett, A. (2005) *Untold Stories*. Faber and Faber.

Bernlef, J. (1984) *Hersenschimmen*. Reprinted (1988) as *Out of Mind* (trans. A. Dixon). Faber and Faber.

Durrant, S. (2000) Serial thinker. *The Guardian*, 24 February (http://www.guardian.co.uk/books/2000/feb/24/kosovo.politics).

Grant, L. (1998) *Remind Me Who I Am, Again*. Granta Books.

Hachinski, V. C., Lassen, N. A. & Marshall, J. (1974) Multi-infarct dementia. A cause of mental deterioration in the elderly. *Lancet*, **2**, 207–210.

Harpham, W. S. & Hoel, D. (1997) Raising the curtain on cancer. Is the puzzle finally becoming clear? *Postgraduate Medicine*, **102**, 232–236.

Ignatieff, M. (1993) *Scar Tissue*. Chatto & Windus.

Taylor, D. J. (2003) They knew her too well. *The Guardian*, 26 August (http://www.guardian.co.uk/books/2003/aug/26/biography.irismurdoch).

Wilson, A. N. (2003) *Iris as I knew Her*. Hutchinson.

CHAPTER 10

Portrayal of intellectual disability in fiction

Anupama Iyer

Outside the sphere of medical and social care people with intellectual disability (also known as learning disability in UK health services) represent a statistical minority. Few people have first-hand experience of knowing or living with someone who has an intellectual disability. Despite this, most people do hold an image of what a person with intellectual disability looks like. This image is partly based on how people with intellectual disability are depicted in fiction and by the media. This depiction both shapes and reflects how society views such individuals.

Parallels exist between literary depictions of intellectual disability and of mental illness. In describing Bertha Mason in *Jane Eyre* (1847), Charlotte Bronte drew upon a popular 19th-century stereotype of madness. At the time, the notion that a madwoman should be feared and loathed, shut away from polite society and beyond cure, was hardly contested. Since then, subjective yet fictional accounts of mental illness such as Sylvia Plath's *The Bell Jar* (1963) have contributed to a redefinition of mental illness (see Oyebode: Chapter 4, this volume).

Intellectual disability is fundamentally different in this respect because its very nature makes it difficult or impossible for people with the condition to write about what it is like to live with it. They are unable to contribute to the discourse by either contesting or confirming their portrayal. Fiction is a case in point; it is a medium to which persons with intellectual disabilities have little or no access yet it is a ready source of their portrayal.

One of the goals of a novelist is to create images that are coherent and believable. The best fiction draws vivid pictures that leave readers feeling that they know what they have probably never seen. However, that is seldom the novelist's main aim. The novel tells a story, creating tension and momentum through actions of characters that drive forward the narrative shape of the plot. Thus, in a novel that includes an individual with intellectual disability, the author will reflect not only what they know about intellectual disabilities as a condition, but also what they want the character to do within the story. In this project only the relevant facets of the character are highlighted. Although the author broadly reflects what is culturally accepted about the condition of the character, they are not obliged to be either medically accurate or morally balanced in their description.

Thus, we are left with a situation in which the author may present, quite legitimately, truths, half-truths or complete fiction which the reader may in good faith take to be facts. Owing to fiction's reach, these images are then likely to further shape how people with intellectual disability are viewed by society.

The fact that the reader will probably have had limited direct experience of the portrayal and that the person portrayed has little or no control over this depiction presents unique ethical considerations. A reader with little experience of intellectual disability in real life has no opportunity for the corrective influence of close contact, so the images created may take on a life of their own, growing and intensifying without check. There is the additional danger that this may increase the distance between the representation and the object of interest: the portraiture may degenerate into a hall of mirrors, in which images and impressions are endlessly recycled and distorted.

The depiction of intellectual disability in itself presents certain technical challenges. These challenges may be variously overcome by employing first-person narratives or by description of appearance and observable behaviour.

Subjective accounts

Descriptions of people with intellectual disability written in the first person are relatively rare in fiction. There are inherent difficulties in fashioning a convincing internal voice for a character whose life and experiences the author cannot share. This difficulty of putting oneself in the shoes of a character whose situation is foreign to the author is usually overcome in fiction by the narrator's empathy for what it might be like to be that character. Alternatively, the author aims at achieving a very high degree of technical accuracy in describing the character's behaviour and environment.

However, both techniques present difficulties. For authors relying on their own empathy, intellectual disability poses a fundamental paradox: when writers 'speak' for a character with intellectual disability they essentially use their creative intelligence to construct both an inner and an outer world view for a character defined by intellectual limitations, a situation they do not share. For those using the descriptive technique, it is often difficult to maintain logical consistency in what the character can do, say and think. This is true even of the most sympathetic portrayals based on real-life models when the author has no way of checking beyond observable behaviour.

Intellectual disability in a sense is always seen from the outside. The technique of describing behaviours from which motives are inferred is commonly used in fiction, particularly in the crime genre, and it assumes a degree of congruence of thoughts and feelings between the reader and the character. The reader is expected to think that the behaviour described indicates (signifies) certain thoughts or mood states. Shifty eyes indicate something to hide, a stutter signifies something unsaid. In applying the same rule to people with intellectual disability, the author assumes rather than knows such things to be true. In fact, shifty eyes may be indicative of muscle weakness, and a stutter may be neurological in origin: a person with intellectual disability is unable to explain this. Consequently, intellectual disability is forever seen from the outside.

Both the difficulties and successes of these methods of depiction are best exemplified in the character of Benjy Compson in William Faulkner's *The Sound and The Fury* (1929). The novel about the Compson family in the American South is organised into four sections. In the first of these, the narrator is Benjy, a 33-year-old man who has a mental age of 3 (profound intellectual disability). The second section is narrated by Quentin, who is depicted as insane, the third by Jason, who is sane but affectionless. The fourth (with a third-person narrator), centres on the figure of Dilsey, the Black servant who represents the voice of endurance and stability.

The character of Benjy is unique because we hear him speak before we see him as others do. We engage with Benjy's world from the inside, and are called on to provide coherence and meaning to the narrative that Benjy himself cannot provide.

Benjy's narrative is diffuse and chaotic: events seem to coalesce, characters to wander in and out. It is only when the novel unfolds that we realise how much of the narrative Faulkner manages to convey through Benjy's inchoate impressions. Benjy has difficulties with the concept of time because of his intellectual disability. His impressions are a mixture of the immediate and the past. He is unable to separate ongoing experience from distant memory, and because of this the whole of his 33 years reads like the unclouded present.

Benjy's descriptions are primarily based on what he perceives with his senses. This is vividly illustrated in his version of a ride in a horse-drawn carriage: 'I could *hear*[1] Queenie's feet and the *bright shapes* went *smooth and steady* on both sides, the *shadows* of them following across Queenie's back' (Faulkner,1978 reprint: p. 9).

This description is based on sight and sound. Its meaning becomes obvious only when Faulkner himself renders it into recognisable images in the closing paragraphs of the book: 'Queenie moved again [...] her feet began to clip-clop steadily again [...] at once Benjy hushed [...] the cornice and the façade flowed from left to right, post and tree, window and doorway and signboard, each in its ordered place' (p. 321).

---

1 Italics in quotations are my own, used to highlight aspects of the thesis

In Benjy's undifferentiated universe sensations are shown to merge: 'I couldn't see it [his sister's slipper] but my hands saw it and I could hear it getting night. [...] I could see the window where the trees were buzzing' (pp. 70, 73).

Benjy's lack of conceptual schemas is deliberately contrasted with the distorted schemas of Quentin's insanity. Benjy is unable to differentiate between deliberate actions of living beings from events in the inanimate world. This lack of higher-order processing is also reflected in his inability to attribute motives and meaning to his interactions with others. He describes an emotive interchange between himself and Dilsey in bland, concrete terms: 'She gave me a flower and her hand went away' (p. 8).

Events just seem to happen to him and around him. He is unable to separate the incidental from the intentional, the important from the trivial. Despite this, Benjy seems to have an almost instinctive grasp of primary emotions. He feels what he cannot know or name. He is unable to account for Mrs Patterson's distress when her husband intercepts her clandestine correspondence but readily recognises the emotion in this situation:

> Mr. Patterson was chopping in the green flowers. Mrs Patterson came across the garden running [...] When I saw her eyes, I began to cry [...] Give it to me. Quick [...] Mr Patterson came fast, with the hoe. She was trying to climb the fence [...] He took the letter [...] I saw her eyes again and I ran down the hill (pp. 11–12).

His own emotions however, are expressed in concrete physical terms. His love and longing for his sister Caddy are conveyed through his pre-occupation with her slipper. Faulkner describes to great effect Benjy's comfort in inanimate objects such as cushions and flowers and his distress when these are taken from him. Benjy's need for sameness is vividly evoked in the closing passages of the book, when he is shown to be very disturbed by the change in the direction of his routine drive around the Confederacy Statue.

In describing these precise minutiae of behaviour, Faulkner uses his observations of Benjy's real-life model to great effect (Halliwell, 2004). He manages to convey the purity of Benjy's sensate universe despite the reader's misgivings about someone with a mental age of 3 speaking fluently, in perfect syntax, perceiving things he could not possibly perceive. Despite these logical inconsistencies the reader is carried along by the power of the narrative voice. The reader ignores, in complicity, the fact that Faulkner's intelligence can never speak for Benjy's lack of it.

Physical description

Describing the physical form of a character with intellectual disability has the advantage of making concrete the abstract concept of the disability: a character who cannot be heard must be seen. It also plays on the often unspoken assumption that people are as people look. This belief is so widespread that people with visible anomalies are often assumed to be intellectually disabled, even if they are not.

Harper Lee in *To Kill a Mocking Bird* (1960) describes Boo Radley as:

> about six feet tall, judging by his tracks; he dined on raw squirrels and any cats he could catch, that's why his hands were blood-stained – if you ate an animal raw you could never wash the blood off. There was a long jagged scar that ran down his face; what teeth he had were yellow and rotten, his eyes popped, and he drooled most of the time (Lee, 1997 reprint: p. 14).

Mannerisms and accessories are used to further demarcate individuals with intellectual disability from other people. Charles Dickens in his novel *Barnaby Rudge* (1840–41) uses Barnaby's clothes to emphasise his difference:

> His dress was of green, *clumsily* trimmed here and there – apparently by his own hands with gaudy lace [...] He had ornamented his hat with a cluster of peacock's feathers, but they were limp and broken, and now trailed negligently down his back [...] The *fluttered and confused disposition* of all the motley scraps that formed his dress, bespoke [...] *the disorder of his mind* (Dickens, 1998 reprint: p. 28).

Resemblance to and kinship with animals is often called forth to emphasise the difference of people with intellectual disability or to signal that they are not quite human. In *Of Mice and Men* (1937), Steinbeck describes Lennie as 'a huge man, shapeless of face with large pale eyes [...] he walked heavily, dragging his feet a little, the way a bear drags his paws' [Steinbeck, 2000 reprint: p. 4]. The almost otherworldly kinship with animals is also used time and again. Barnaby speaks of his pet raven almost as he would of another person: 'He takes such care of me besides! [...] He watches all the time I sleep, he practices his new learning softly' (Dickens, 1998 reprint: p. 131).

Eccentricity suggestive of autism seems to go hand in hand with visible anomalies. Even if we take into account the relatively higher rates of autistic-spectrum disorders in intellectual disability, it is remarkable how many authors use this facet of eccentricity disproportionately often to depict characters with intellectual disabilities. Hilary Dickinson (2000) has suggested that the use of eccentricity shields the reader from what she deems the 'literary inelegance' of intellectual disability. Eccentricity and autistic traits confer what she calls 'stylishness' that intellectual disability is seen as lacking.

Eccentricity suggests mysterious, often spiritual, gifts and exotic possibilities. Joseph Conrad uses this in emphasising the spiritual aspects of Stevie, a character with intellectual disability in *The Secret Agent* (1907), describing him as:

> drawing circles, circles, innumerable circles, concentric, eccentric, coruscating whirl of circles that by their tangled multitude of repeated curves, uniformity of form, and confusion of intersecting lines [...] suggested a rendering of cosmic chaos, the symbolism of the mad art attempting the inconceivable (Conrad, 1996 reprint: p. 46).

119

In addition to making the individual stand out visually, eccentricity and anomaly also serve the psychological function of distancing the intellectually disabled figure from the reader. Gilman (1988) proposes that in fiction disabled characters are overwhelmingly cast as the 'other'. In signalling their difference, the author protects readers from the fear that the character described could possibly be them.

Behavioural descriptions

The casting of the intellectually disabled figure as the 'other' is also achieved by calling on distinctive mannerisms and nuances of behaviour. In *Barnaby Rudge*, Barnaby's exaggerated mannerisms serve to highlight his difference in the same way as his eccentric attire: 'He nodded – not once or twice, but a score of times, and that with a *fantastic exaggeration* which would have kept his head in motion for an hour' (Dickens, 1998 reprint: p. 27). Steinbeck uses the simple act of drinking to signal Lennie's disabilities, in this passage from *Of Mice and Men* (1937): '[Lennie] *flung* himself down and drank [...] with *long gulps snorting into the water like a horse*' (Steinbeck, 2000 reprint: p.4). Conrad uses Stevie's motor restlessness to convey the fear and perplexity that are a part of his psyche: 'A brusque question caused him to stutter to the point of suffocation. When startled by anything perplexing he used to squint horribly' (Conrad, 1996 reprint: p. 17). Rohinton Mistry in *Such a Long Journey* (1991) uses his character Tehmul's distinctive speech to describe him:

> the words of Tehmul-Lungraa's abbreviated vocabulary always emerged at breakneck speed, whizzing incomprehensibly past the listener's ears [...]. Tehmul's cascading utterances were always bereft of commas, exclamation marks, semi-colons, question marks: all swept away. [...] The verbal velocity only allowed for the use of the full stop. And it was not really a full stop [...] rather, a minimal halt anywhere he chose to re-oxygenate his lungs [p. 31].
>
> GustadGustadrunningrace.fastfast.chicken first [p. 32].

Tehmul has other behaviours that intensely annoy adults, including following people, and scratching his loins and armpits.

Motives are attributed and causes are inferred regarding the person through the medium of such mannerisms, which may be partly or purely involuntary. For instance, Steinbeck accurately describes Lennie's echopraxia, which he chooses to interpret as indicative of Lennie's blind idolisation of George. However, echopraxia may in this case be neurologically hard wired and not open to easy meaningful interpretation: 'Lennie who had been watching imitated George exactly. He pushed himself back, drew his knees, [...] looked over to George to see whether he had it just right. He pulled his hat down a little more over his eyes, the way George's hat was' (Steinbeck, 2000 reprint: p.5). Similarly, stuttering, a speech impediment not limited to people with intellectual disability, is used by Conrad to signify Stevie's hesitant personhood.

Authors may also choose to focus on lack of normative social functioning. For instance, Conrad calls on Stevie's inability to keep down a basic job to characterise him: 'as an errand boy he did not turn out a great success. He forgot his messages; he was easily diverted from the straight path of duty by the attractions of strangers and dogs [...] by the comedies of the street which he contemplated open-mouthed' (Conrad, 1996 reprint: p. 17). Alternatively, unusual occupations are highlighted, as in the case of Tehmul, who for a nominal fee disposes of rats caught by other tenants of his building. Some of these behaviours are attributed to specific aetiologies, which are used to further define what a character does.

Drawing on the theories of causation

Authors usually make an effort to account for the intellectual disabilities of their characters. This aetiology varies widely depending on cultural notions, prevalent medical theories and, perhaps most importantly, the thrust of the narrative.

In *Barnaby Rudge*, Dickens evokes the supernatural in describing the cause of Barnaby's intellectual disability: 'They recollected how the change had come [on Barnaby's mother] and could call to mind that when the son was born, upon the very day the deed was known, he bore upon his wrist what seemed a smear of blood but half washed out' (Dickens, 1998 reprint: p. 41). In contrast, in the character of Maggy in *Little Dorrit* (1855–57) he creates a medically accurate portrait. Traces of the encephalopathic origins of her intellectual disability are visible in her dyspraxia and echolalic, fragmented speech (Dickinson, 2000). Dickens introduces Maggy into the narrative as follows:

> an excited figure of a strange kind bounced against them[...] fell down, and scattered the contents of a large basket, filled with potatoes[...] and she then began to pick up the potatoes[...] Maggy *picked up very few potatoes, and a great quantity of mud.*
> 'This is Maggy, Sir.'
> '*Maggy, Sir*', echoed the personage presented.
> ⋮
> 'You can't *think how good she is, Sir', said Little Dorrit.*
> '*Good* she is' echoed Maggy [Dickens, 1996 reprint: p. 97].

Less than two decades separate these depictions, but there is a significant difference in what Dickens wants these characters to do within the narratives. In *Barnaby Rudge*, he chooses to link Barnaby's affinities with the natural world to a supernatural cause, whereas in *Little Dorrit* the focus is firmly on Maggy as a patient recipient of Little Dorrit's nurturing.

The various ways in which the aetiology of the disabilities is used within the plot is illustrated particularly well in the character of Sufiya Zinobia. Salman Rushdie in *Shame* (1983) mixes both mystical and medical aetiologies to account for Sufiya Zinobia's developmental difficulties. Her mother turns to the local doctor to cure Sufiya's brain fever:

> a local hakim prepared an expensive liquid distilled from cactus roots, ivory dust and parrot feathers [...] [which] had the unfortunate side-effect of slowing her down for the rest of her years [...] because the unfortunate side-effect of a potion so filled with the elements of longevity was to retard the progress of time inside the body of anyone to whom it was given [p. 100].

Here the theory chosen is not a reflection of prevailing medical ideas regarding intellectual disabilities; rather it feeds the magical aura that Rushdie wants to create around his character's supernatural powers.

The aetiology chosen can also reflect the fate of characters and can be used to justify other protagonists' interest in them. For example, in *Such a Long Journey* Tehmul's developmental disabilities are attributed to traumatic brain injury but also to neglected education. This serves to minimise his otherness and makes Gustad's interest in him understandable.

Social causes are also used to signal possibilities for rehabilitation and change. This is in sharp contrast to narratives in which developmental disabilities are attributed to genetic degeneration and miscegenation, where no such change is possible. This issue is cogently argued in the *Secret Agent*, where a character evokes Lombroso's theories of genetic degeneration to account for Stevie's intellectual disability. He is robustly contradicted by another character, an anarchist, who emphasises the role of society.

What function does the depiction serve?

At the most literal level, the depiction serves to drive the narrative forward. However, characters with intellectual disability have seldom been depicted as active agents with motives and volition, even when central to the narrative. They do not initiate important events: things happen to them or through them.

In Dickens's historical tale about the Gordon Riots of 1780, the eponymous Barnaby Rudge is shown as a passive participant in events that nearly lead to his hanging. He joins the rioters to wear their uniform and carry their flag. Dickens describes how Barnaby marches with the other rioters: 'forgetful of all things in the ecstasy of the moment [...] heedless of the weight of the great banner [...] mindful only of its flashing in the sun and rustling in the summer breeze, on he went [...] *the only light-hearted, undesigning creature* in the whole assembly' (Dickens, 1998 reprint: pp. 371–372). Afterwards 'He had *no consciousness* [...] *of having done wrong* [...] *no new perceptions in the merit of the cause'* (pp. 528–529).

Far from being active protagonists, characters with intellectual disability are often portrayed as passive victims of exploitation. For instance, in *Such a Long Journey* Tehmul is used as a receptacle for spells to reverse the ill-fortunes plaguing the protagonist Gustad's household. Ms Kutpitia, the local herbalist in the novel, has very few scruples in casting the spell on Tehmul. She convinces Gustad's reluctant wife by saying: 'How much brain does he have to begin with [...] so what difference will it make [...] Tehmul himself will not notice anything. What I say is that we should be happy that for the first time he will do something good for another person' (Mistry, 1991: p. 110).

When given affection it is never expected that intellectually disabled characters can or may reciprocate. In *Shame*, Sufiya Zinobia's father and governess show her affection with no expectation of a return.

Characters with intellectual disability are often the butt of ridicule and casual cruelty. Such cruelty may even come from a caregiver, as described poignantly in *Of Mice and Men*. Lennie's friend and protector George brags about Lennie's devotion to him, saying:

> 'Why he'd do any damn thing I tol' him to [...] One day a bunch of guys was standin' around up on the Sacramento River [...] I was feeling pretty smart [...] I turns to Lennie and says "Jump in". An' he jumps in [...] couldn't swim a stroke. He damn near drowned before we could get him. An' he was so damn nice to me for pullin' 'im out. Clean forgot I told 'im to jump in' [Steinbeck, 2000 reprint: p. 41].

People with intellectual disability are often depicted as being unable to regulate their sexual and aggressive drives. Tehmul displays an unreasoning cruelty in disposing of the rats:

> A bucket of water was filled and the rats ducked one by one. He pulled them out before the end, gasping and suffocating, and kept on till he was bored with the game, or a *miscalculation* drowned the rats. Sometimes for variety, he boiled a large kettle of water [...] he poured the boiling water a little at a time. As the rats squealed and writhed in agony, he watched their reaction with great interest, particularly their tails, proud of the pretty colours he could bestow on them [Mistry, 1991: p. 33].

Sufiya Zinobia is shown to internalise the hate and rage as self harm:

> [she would] tear each damaged hair in two, all the way down to the roots. She did this seriously, systematically. Her eyes, while she worked, acquired a dull glint, a gleam of distant ice or fire from far below their habitually opaque surface; and the torn cloud of hair stood around her face and formed in the sunlight a kind of halo of destruction [Rushdie, 1983: p. 136].

The association of intellectual disability with violence is so prevalent that characters with intellectual disabilities are often invested with a sinister aura without really having to do anything.

In her description of Boo Radley (1960), Harper Lee uses the voice of the child narrator Scout to spell out this recognised stereotype:

> Inside the house lived a malevolent phantom [...] people said he went out at night when the moon was high and peeped in windows. When people's azaleas froze in a cold snap, it was because he had breathed on them. Once the town was terrorized by a series of morbid nocturnal events: people's chickens and pets were found mutilated: although the culprit was crazy Eddie [...] people still looked at Radley Place, unwilling to discard their suspicions [Lee, 1997 reprint: p. 9].

123

Boo does very little and typically we hear more about him than from him in the novel. The myth of his malevolence is never contested.

Use of characters with intellectual disability as a narrative device

In essence, writers employ figures with intellectual disability either as a passive narrative device, or as contrasts to the other characters.

Barnaby Rudge's innocence is a foil to the rioters' rage and complex political motives. Boo Radley is a foil to another marginalised group in the story: Black people in the American South. Tehmul's simple life in the here and now is in contrast to Gustad's agonised search for meaning. Stevie's blind loyalty is a mirror to the corruption and inept plotting of the anarchists who set him up.

When used as a counterpoint, such characters become avolitional receptacles of various abstract qualities that the author ascribes to them. These symbolic qualities assume centre stage and displace the human aspects of the figures.

What do the characters with intellectual disability symbolise?

Lennie, Stevie and Barnaby are all symbols of a lyrical innocence, untouched by worldly reason. This is reflected in Barnaby's return to his idyllic rural home: 'He lived with his mother on the farm [...] he was known to every bird or beast about the place and had a name for everyone. Never was there [...] a creature more popular with the young or old, a blither or more happy soul than Barnaby' (Dickens, 1998 reprint: p. 634). This child-like innocence is highlighted by the characters' rapport with animals, which reflects that they are closer to nature than to man. This is seen in Lennie's feeling for mice, Stevie's sympathy for cart horses, Barnaby's affection for his raven and Tehmul's delight in things that fly. This symbolism is inverted when the cruelty or sexual disinhibition of an intellectually disabled character are emphasised. Intellectual disability then comes to represent dysregulation and destruction unchecked by reason.

In *Shame*, Sufiya Zinobia alternates between these two symbolisms. As 'Sufiya the Saint' she 'suffers in our stead' (Rushdie, 1983: p. 141), becoming a voiceless symbol for the disenfranchised. As 'Sufiya the Beast' she uses her superhuman powers to decapitate four young men and comes to represent the aggressive powers of unreason. Her use as a symbol does not allow her to be ordinary. She is either less than human or superhuman.

It has been suggested that Benjy's developmental disability 'is a symptom of the decline of his family and culture' (Halliwell, 2004: p. 20). Benjy as a person becomes a metonymy for the 'moral decay of the Compson family' (Halliwell, 2004: p. 20).

These symbolisms derive some of their power from being subliminal. They are not overtly stated and thus never consciously examined. They perpetuate unspoken stereotypes about intellectual disability. In doing so, they serve to minimise the identity of intellectually disabled people as ordinary individuals and undermine their lived experience.

Even when the images have positive connotations, they are often used to minimise and gloss over real situations in the real world. When portrayed as symbols and stereotypes, people with intellectual disability are not allowed the dignity of ordinary abilities, difficulties and assets. Instead their disability bears what Susan Sontag (1983) calls 'the metaphorical and symbolic weight' of the images assigned to them.

A character with an intellectual disability becomes a silent Rorschach inkblot onto which society projects its desires through the agency of the author.

What would constitute an 'ethical' representation?

The issue of ethical representation of disabilities has been discussed at length by Thomas Couser (2005). He does not advocate a 'positive' image of individuals with disability 'overcoming' their impairments. He suggests instead reasonable precautions that may be exercised in descriptions. He also suggests consultation where possible with people who themselves have the disability: 'Nothing about Us without Us' (Charlton, 1998). In the absence of this individual voice, he recommends that authors:

- consult advocacy or support groups to minimise the possible harm of the representation
- do not depict people with disabilities as 'alien', albeit they may be 'different'
- avoid making one particular trait the overarching, defining facet of the individual
- avoid symbolism that generates set, stereotyped images
- avoid moral attributions to what is, in effect, a part medical (impairment), part social (disability) condition
- acknowledge that disability is the concern not just of the individual but of the world in which that individual is living.

It may be argued that Couser's recommendations may better serve journalists than creators of narratives. However, they are cautionary rather than prescriptive. The desire for an uncluttered creative space needs to be balanced against not harming a vulnerable group.

Conclusion

Fictional images significantly influence how people with intellectual disabilities are viewed by society. This inevitably affects the lives of these individuals and of the people who care for them. Knowledge of fictional images enhances clinicians' understanding of individual lives. It also raises awareness of the unspoken stereotypes that exist in popular culture regarding people with disabilities as a group. This may prove to be a valuable tool for reasoned and informed advocacy when clinicians speak for or about persons with intellectual disabilities.

References

Bronte, C. (1847) *Jane Eyre*. Reprinted 1996. Penguin.

Charlton, J. I. (1998) *Nothing about Us without Us: Disability, Oppression and Empowerment*. University of California Press.

Conrad, J. (1907) *The Secret Agent*. Reprinted 1996. Penguin.

Couser, G. T. (2005) Paradigms' cost: representing vulnerable subjects. *Literature and Medicine*, **24** (1), 19–30.

Dickens, C. (1840–41) *Barnaby Rudge*. Reprinted 1998. Wordsworth Classics.

Dickens, C. (1855–57) *Little Dorrit*. Reprinted 1996. Wordsworth Classics.

Dickinson, H. (2000) Idiocy in nineteenth century fiction compared with medical perspectives of the time. *History of Psychiatry*, **11**, 291–309.

Faulkner, W. (1929) *The Sound and the Fury*. Reprinted 1978. Chatto and Windus.

Gilman, S. L. (1988) *Disease and Representation: Images of Sickness from Madness to AIDS*. Cornell University Press.

Halliwell, M. (2004) *Images of Idiocy: The Idiot Figure in Modern Fiction and Film*. Ashgate Publishing.

Lee, H. (1960) *To Kill a Mocking Bird*. Reprinted 1997. Arrow Books.

Mistry, R. (1991) *Such a Long Journey*. Chatto and Windus.

Plath, S. (1963) *The Bell Jar*. Faber and Faber.

Rushdie, S. (1983) *Shame*. Jonathan Cape.

Sontag, S. (1983) *Illness as Metaphor*. Penguin.

Steinbeck, J. (1937) *Of Mice and Men*. Reprinted 2000. Penguin Classics.

CHAPTER 11

Autism in fiction and autobiography

Gordon Bates

Modern Western literature and popular culture are littered with stereotypes of some of the facets of autism and Asperger syndrome, despite their relatively recent description in the scientific literature. Leo Kanner and Hans Asperger made their original separate descriptions of the conditions as recently as the early 1940s (Kanner, 1943; Asperger, 1944), but many recognisably autistic characters pre-date this.

Literary depictions range from the reserved, emotionless intellectuals typified by Conan Doyle's Sherlock Holmes, who first appeared in publication in 1887, to the guileless *faux naifs* whose role in the narrative is to act as a mirror to the social mores or the inequities of the world around them. Examples of these innocents include Melville's Bartleby, in *Bartleby, The Scrivener: A Story of Wall Street* (1853) and Harper Lee's Boo Radley in *To Kill a Mocking Bird* (1960). Other aspects of the autistic personality are a rich source of humour in comic writing, from the pompous and pedantic Mr Pooter in the Grossmiths' *Diary of a Nobody* (1892) to the grotesque Ignatius P. Reilly in J. K. Toole's *A Confederacy of Dunces* (1980). However, novels containing characters who show the full triad of primary symptoms of autistic disorder, with impairment of language and socialising and a preference for routine, remain relatively rare (Box 11.1).

The recent growth in rates of diagnosis and the explosion of popular interest in autism in general and in Asperger syndrome in particular have led to an increase in more complete and accurate depictions and the flowering of the so-called autie-biography (Box 11.2). These accounts also mark a change in societal views towards those with autism, who are increasingly seen not in voiceless supporting roles or bit parts but as characters in their own right.

In this chapter, I shall primarily use extracts from two of the most influential of the recent books to illustrate features of the conditions and highlight the novelty and originality of the autistic-spectrum world view. My first example is the popular work of fiction, *The Curious Incident of the Dog in the Night-Time* (Haddon, 2003), in which a teenage boy with Asperger syndrome discovers more than he bargains for when he investigates the

---

Box 11.1 A selection of fictional works containing characters with explicit autism

The Curious Incident of the Dog in the Night-Time (by Mark Haddon): Christopher Boone

The Speed of Dark (by Elizabeth Moon): Lou Arrendale

The Minotaur (by Barbara Vine): John Cosway

Martian Time-Slip (by Philip K. Dick): Manfred Steiner

Little Green Man (by Simon Armitage): Travis

Clear Light of Day (by Anita Desai): Baba

Family Pictures (by Sue Miller): Randall Eberhardt

---

murder of his neighbour's dog. Temple Grandin's autobiography *Emergence: Labeled Autistic* (Grandin & Scariano, 1986) is my second example. Temple Grandin has written several subsequent books and has lectured widely about her experiences. She has become an expert in animal handling and continues to pursue a university career. In her book, she describes her continuing struggle with social understanding which leads to her expulsion from mainstream school but her eventual redemption, becoming a university academic. This early text has paved the way for other writers with autism, young and old, to tell their stories.

Michael Fitzgerald (2005) has argued that many literary greats themselves had autism and that much of their talent is tied in with their condition. This may seem unlikely, given that language impairment is part of the condition,

---

Box 11.2 Books by people with autism and by carers

Emergence: Labelled Autistic and *Thinking in Pictures* by Temple Grandin

Nobody Nowhere: The Remarkable Autobiography of an Autistic Girl by Donna Williams

Freaks, Geeks and Asperger's Syndrome: A User Guide to Adolescence by Luke Jackson

Martian in the Playground: Understanding the Schoolchild with Asperger's Syndrome by Claire Sainsbury

Carers' accounts:

George and Sam by Charlotte Moore

Exiting Nirvana: A Daughter's Life with Autism by Clara Claiborne Park

---

but perhaps it accounts for their originality of voice. Other critics have also questioned whether those with Asperger syndrome have the levels of empathy required to meet the needs of the reading public. Fitzgerald cites Hans Asperger's observation that children with autistic psychopathy develop 'highly grammatical speech and they may be uncommonly apt at using experiences coined spontaneously' (Asperger, 1974). He also suggests that as social outsiders with great powers of observation, writers with Asperger syndrome can be very objective about the social relationships that form the basis of most novels. He bases his diagnoses on biographical information and concludes that writers such as Jonathan Swift, Herman Melville, Lewis Carroll, Arthur Conan Doyle and George Orwell all fell on the autistic spectrum. The biographical details do suggest that these writers were 'odd' by the standards of the time but ultimately the case is not made that these authors would fulfil diagnostic criteria for Asperger syndrome. Nevertheless, it is worth noting that they penned a couple of the fictional examples already mentioned.

Difference of world view

Writers can use a number of different techniques to convey the sense of difference and distance between the 'neurotypical' (mainstream) and autistic world view. Compare the arresting openings of Temple Grandin's book and Mark Haddon's. Grandin describes a 'flashbulb' memory of a car journey taken with her mother and sister when she was 3 years old. She describes her unwillingness to wear a tight-fitting hat and the lengths to which she went to avoid wearing it:

> I fingered the painful hat, trying to rub away the walls of fabric. Humming tunelessly, I massaged the material over and over. Now the hat lay in my lap like an ugly blue blob. I had to get rid of it. I decided to throw it out the window. Mother wouldn't notice. She was too busy driving. But at a little over three years old I couldn't crank my window down. Now the hat felt hot and prickly on my lap. It lay there waiting like a monster. Impulsively I leaned forward and tossed it out Mother's window.
> She yelled. I covered my ears to shut out the hurting sound. She made a grab for the hat. The car swerved. Suddenly we were jolting into the other lane. I leaned back against the seat and enjoyed the jostling. Jean was in the back seat crying. Even today I remember the bushes planted along the highway. I close my eyes and feel again the warm sun streaming through the window, smell the exhaust fumes and see the red tractor-trailer truck come closer and closer.
> Mother tried to turn the wheel, but it was too late. I heard the crush of metal and felt a violent jolt as we sideswiped the red tractor-trailer truck and sud-denly stopped. I yelled, 'Ice.Ice.Ice.' as broken glass showered all over me. I was not scared at all. It was kind of exciting [Grandin & Scariano, 1986: p. 17].

In *The Curious Incident of the Dog in the Night-Time* we meet our hero Christopher Boone in a similarly striking introduction:

> I pulled the fork out of the dog and lifted him into my arms and hugged him. He was leaking blood from the fork-holes.

I like dogs. You always know what a dog is thinking. It has four moods. Happy, sad, cross and concentrating. Also, dogs are faithful and they do not tell lies because they cannot talk.

I had been hugging the dog for 4 minutes when I heard screaming. I looked up and saw Mrs Shears running towards me from the patio. She was wearing pyjamas and a housecoat. Her toenails were painted bright pink and she had no shoes on.

She was shouting, 'What in fuck's name have you done to my dog?'

I do not like people shouting at me. It makes me scared that they are going to hit me or touch me and I do not know what is going to happen.

'Let go of the dog,' she shouted. 'Let go of the fucking dog for Christ's sake.'

I put the dog down on the lawn and moved back 2 metres.

She bent down. I thought she was going to pick the dog up herself, but she didn't. Perhaps she noticed how much blood there was and didn't want to get dirty. Instead, she started screaming again.

I put my hands over my ears and closed my eyes and rolled forward till I was hunched up with my forehead pressed onto the grass. The grass was wet and cold. It was nice [Haddon, 2003: p. 4].

Both books are written in the first person, which forces you to share their autistic world view. They are deliberately written in simple child-like language, with its associations of innocence and naivety. In the second extract the use of language is stilted: 'leaking blood' for bleeding. In both extracts the emotional response of the narrator is disturbingly out of kilter with our expectations of how children should react to the events that are portrayed. Both writers fail to focus on the distressing experience of the events and either describe no emotional response or a seemingly inappropriate one. The matter-of-fact tone and the emphasis on irrelevant visual details also alerts us to the fact that the narrator is 'unreliable'. We learn at the outset that we will have to reinterpret their perceptions and version of events as their account is so highly subjective. Mark Haddon makes use of dramatic irony throughout, ensuring through his descriptions that the reader understands more about what is going on than Christopher himself does.

Social impairment

Humans are such social creatures that those who do not need company or do not display emotion in culturally sanctioned ways are viewed with suspicion. Such schizoid characters usually come to a bad end. Consider the fate of Mersault in Albert Camus' *L'Étranger* (usually translated as *The Stranger* or *The Outsider*) (1942). When he kills a young Algerian man, he is viewed as more culpable for being seemingly unaffected by the recent death of his mother than for the murder itself.

Although some with autism are self-absorbed and content with their own company, many with Asperger syndrome are keen for social contact but struggle to mix or to maintain friendships. Problems with empathising appear to be at the core of this. It is a great handicap being unable to infer other people's emotions from their nonverbal communication or the immediate context.

In *The Curious Incident of the Dog in the Night-Time*, there is a scene which illustrates Christopher's lack of empathy in a particularly poignant manner. In the course of the book, Christopher discovers that his mother left his father for another man, but his father had lied about her death. This is the moment of their reunion:

> And she said, 'Why didn't you write to me, Christopher? I wrote you all those letters. I kept thinking something dreadful had happened, or you'd moved away and I'd never find out where you were.'
> And I said, 'Father said you were dead.'
> And she said, 'What?'
> And I said, 'He said you went into hospital because you had something wrong with your heart. And then you had a heart attack and died and he kept all the letters in a shirt box in the cupboard in his bedroom and I found them because I was looking for a book I was writing about Wellington being killed and he'd taken it away from me and hidden it in the shirt box.'
> And then Mother said, 'Oh my God.'
> And then she didn't say anything for a long while. And then she made a loud wailing noise like an animal on a nature programme on television.
> And I didn't like her doing this because it was a loud noise, and I said, 'Why are you doing that?'
> And she didn't say anything for a while, and then she said, 'Oh, Christopher, I'm so sorry.'
> And I said, 'Its not your fault.'
> And then she said, 'Bastard, The bastard.'
> And then, after a while, she said, 'Christopher, let me hold your hand. Just for once. Just for me. Will you? I won't hold it hard,' and she held out her hand.
> And I said, 'I don't like people holding my hand.'
> And then she took her hand back and she said, 'No. OK. That's OK.'
> [Haddon, 2003: p. 236].

Another aspect of poor empathy skills is a lack of self-awareness. If you cannot pick up others' cues, you cannot know how you are being perceived. This results in a lack of restraint that is an important component of many comedic creations. By no means do all such characters have autism, but I believe that one of my favourite characters does. Ignatius J. Reilly is the antihero of *A Confederacy of Dunces* (Toole, 1980). He is a corpulent, flatulent but highly educated and eloquent unemployed man who lives with his mother. He is arrogant and highly judgemental and critical of others. The story revolves around his attempts to get a job at his mother's insistence. This is a very traumatic time for most families with autistic children who have grown up. In the novel, it is a device that brings Ignatius into contact with people he cannot understand and detests. The novel does not mock Ignatius despite his faults; instead the reader sympathises with his plight and his frustration with the idiots around him. In an autistic coincidence, this book gets its title from a Jonathan Swift quotation: 'When a true genius appears in the world, you may know him by this sign, that the dunces are in confederacy against him.'

A green hunting cap squeezed the top of the fleshy balloon of a head. The green earflaps, full of large ears and uncut hair and the fine bristles that grew in the ears themselves, stuck out on either side like turn signals indicating two directions at once. Full, pursed lips protruded beneath the bushy black moustache and, at their corners, sank into little folds of disapproval and potato chip crumbs. In the shadow under the green visor of the cap Ignatius P. Reilly's supercilious blue eyes looked down upon the other people waiting under the clock at the D. H. Holmes department store, studying the crowd of people for bad taste in dress. Several of the outfits, Ignatius noticed, were new enough and expensive enough to be properly considered offenses against taste and decency. Possession of anything new or expensive only reflected a person's lack of theology and geometry; it could even cast doubts upon one's soul.

Ignatius himself was dressed comfortably and sensibly. The hunting cap prevented head colds. The voluminous tweed trousers were durable and permitted unusually free locomotion. Their pleats and nooks contained pockets of warm stale air that soothed Ignatius. The plaid flannel shirt made a jacket unnecessary while the muffler guarded exposed Reilly skin between earflap and collar. The outfit was acceptable by any theological and geometric standards, however abstruse, and suggested a rich inner life [Toole, 2006 reprint: p. 1].

Language use

Oddities in the use of language comprise an important part of the triad of primary autistic symptoms. In life, these peculiarities involve both the form and the content of speech. Mutism, neologisms (novel words) and stock phrases are usually seen in those with autism and learning disability. Literal, pedantic and overly inclusive or formal speech is associated more with Asperger syndrome.

There is a range of ways that these show themselves in life and can be represented in fiction. One of the earliest convincing depictions of adult autism can be found in Herman Melville's short story, *Bartleby, The Scrivener* (1853). The eponymous, mysterious stranger, who comes to work as a copywriter at a New York law firm, is depicted as a tragic but almost noble figure, who dies as a result of his inflexibility. His behaviour is recognisably autistic, with his social aloofness, limited conversational ability and resistance to change. There are additional details which are persuasive. He has restricted food preferences, eating only ginger-nut biscuits. He even has periods of catatonic immobility, first described in relation to autism by Wing & Attwood (1987). Bartleby also has poor eye contact: 'He kept his glance fixed on my bust of Cicero, which as I then sat was directly behind me, some six inches above my head' (Melville, 1990 reprint: p. 19).

The depiction of Bartleby's language also rings true. His language is restricted and stereotyped. He avoids speaking to his work colleagues, but will speak to his supervisor in a limited fashion. His stock phrase is 'I would prefer not to.' He repeats this on 23 occasions in the course of the short story. Even when refusing to do office work he says this phrase in 'a singularly mild, firm voice' so that it is not a challenge. Ironically, this phrase is picked up by his more social co-workers and becomes part of office parlance. Bartleby can be very literal in his understanding of language. After his employer moves to different offices to escape from him, Bartleby remains. When he is asked what he is doing there (in the vacated offices), he replies 'sitting upon the banister'. This is accurate but not the answer to the implied, more general question.

In *The Curious Incident of the Dog in the Night-Time*, there are some well-observed passages of dialogue that illustrate the semantic and pragmatic language problems of those with Asperger syndrome. Semantic impairments refer to the problems in ascertaining meaning from the context when language is ambiguous, whereas pragmatic difficulties are those related to the practicalities of making conversation such as staying on topic and initiating contact.

Christopher starts investigating the death of the dog, like his fictional hero Sherlock Holmes, who in a short story *Silver Blaze* was also struck by 'the curious incident of the dog in the night-time'. Christopher starts by interviewing one of his neighbours:

> So I said, 'Do you know anything about Wellington being killed?'
> And she said, 'I heard about it yesterday. Dreadful. Dreadful.'
> I said, 'Do you know who killed him?'
> And she said, 'No, I don't.'
> I replied, 'Somebody must know because the person who killed Wellington knows that they killed Wellington. Unless they were a mad person and didn't know what they were doing. Or unless they had amnesia.'
> And she said, 'Well, I suppose you're probably right.'
> I said, 'Thank you for helping me with my investigation.'
> And she said, 'You're Christopher, aren't you?'
> I said, 'Yes I live at number 36.'
> And she said, 'We haven't talked before, have we?'
> I said, 'No I don't like talking to strangers. But I'm doing detective work.'
> And she said, 'I see you every day, going to school.'
> I didn't reply to this.
> And she said, 'It's very nice of you to come and say hello.'
> I didn't reply to this either because Mrs Alexander was doing what is called chatting where people say things to each other which aren't questions and answers and aren't connected.
> Then she said, 'Even if it's only because you're doing detective work.'
> And I said, 'Thank you,' again.
> And I was about to turn and walk away when she said, 'I have a grandson your age.'
> I tried to do chatting by saying, 'My age is 15 years and 3 months and 3 days.'
> And she said, 'Well, almost your age.'
> Then we said nothing for a little while until she said, 'You don't have a dog, do you?'
> And I said, 'No'.
> She said, 'You'd probably like a dog, wouldn't you?'
> And I said, 'I have a rat.'
> And she said, 'A rat?'
> And I said, 'He's called Toby.'
> And she said, 'Oh'.

And I said, 'Most people don't like rats because they think they carry diseases like bubonic plague. But that's only because they lived in sewers and stowed away on ships coming from foreign countries where there were strange diseases. But rats are very clean. Toby is always washing himself. And you don't have to take him out for walks. I just let him run around my room so that he gets some exercise. And sometimes he sits on my shoulder or hides in my sleeve like it's a burrow. But rats don't live in burrows in nature.' [Haddon, 2003: p. 50].

Information overload

Sometimes personal accounts and fictions can remind doctors of the more pressing concerns of their patients, helping to shift their clinical focus. Although not a part of the way autistic disorder is defined, those with autism frequently struggle with the processing of sensory information. They can easily be overwhelmed by the sheer mass of information that our senses perpetually generate, particularly at times of stress. They seem to be unable to filter out the extraneous and peripheral. The reverse of this is also true: most of us see but do not see. It is the role of the novelist to help us to observe again.

Several novelists have attempted to encapsulate in literary form the way we think and experience the world continually. Perhaps, the most well known is James Joyce's attempt in *Ulysses* (1922). However, this forbidding book is a considerable challenge to the casual reader. My own preference to exemplify this approach is Nicholson Baker's *The Mezzanine* (1988). The 'action' of this novella takes place in a business lunch hour. It is funny and full of digressions about the minutiae of life such as why plastic straws replaced paper straws despite the fact that they float in fizzy drinks, how to overcome public micturition anxiety and why shoelaces break. The text on the page is deliberately close set. There are few paragraph breaks and almost endless footnotes that go on to the next page. The language is clear but formal, with long rambling sentences containing subclause after subclause. Most striking is the very visual way that the world is described. The descriptions are overinclusive and focus on trade names and seemingly irrelevant details. It has been described as a reflection on the 'Information Age', but I find it very suggestive of the autistic world view, particularly with the fascinating observations about how things work, from everyday objects to body language:

> 'I sign where?'
> 'Anywhere. Here's a pen.'
> I had already half pulled out my shirt-pocket pen, but not wanting to refuse her offer, I hesitated; at the same time she saw that I already had a pen and with an 'Oh' began to retract hers from the proffering position; meanwhile I had decided to accept hers and had let go of the one in my pocket, not registering until it was too late that she had withdrawn her offer; she seeing that I was now beginning to reach for her pen, cancelled her retraction, but meanwhile I, processing her earlier corrective movement, had gone back to reaching for

my own pen – so we went through a little foilwork that was like the mutual bobbings you exchange with an oncoming pedestrian, as both of you lurch to indicate whether you are going to pass to the right or left [Baker, 1990 reprint: p. 30].

Sensory disturbance

Many people with autism find particular sounds, smells and textures so intense that they are painful or distressing. Tony Attwood (1998), a leading figure in the advancement of the popular understanding of autism, describes an evocative extract from the scientific literature (Cesaroni & Garber, 1991). When asked why he was reluctant to play in the garden at home a young boy with autism replied that he hated the 'clack-clack' noise of the wings of butterflies. This is a good example of the usefulness of first-hand accounts of autism in qualitative research but equally a beautifully poetic image.

In *Emergence: Labeled Autistic*, Temple Grandin describes her own problems with sensory modulation and how specific sounds, smells and textures are experienced as unbearable. By describing her sensations at Christmas, she subverts our Western cultural norms of an idealised family Christmas:

> At those times [Christmas and Thanksgiving] our home bulged with relatives. The clamour of many voices, the different smells – perfume, cigars, damp wool caps or gloves – people moving about at different speeds, going in different directions, the constant noise and confusion, the constant touching were overwhelming. One very, very overweight aunt, who was very generous and caring let me use her professional oil paints. I liked her. Still when she hugged me, I was totally engulfed and I panicked. It was like being suffocated by a mountain of marshmallows. I withdrew because her abundant affection overwhelmed my nervous system [Grandin & Scariano, 1986: p. 25].

Autism and society

Some novels have even brought important issues from the culture of autism to a wider audience. In Asperger chat rooms people debate whether or not autism is an illness, a handicap or a condition. In Elizabeth Moon's science fiction novel *The Speed of Dark* (2002), the possibility of a cure for autism is considered and the concept of what constitutes normality is questioned. Owing to his phenomenal ability to see patterns in data-sets the central character, Lou Arrendale, has been head hunted to work for a prestigious company. Like all his immediate colleagues, he has autism and his skills are known to be related to his condition. Their supervisor ensures that they work in an autism-friendly environment and protects them from the prejudices of other employees. Their work environment includes hanging mobiles, a gym, bathroom facilities and a trampoline to bounce away their stresses. The problems come when the new company executives see these things as an expensive luxury and question the need for preferential treatment. They propose experimental 'normalisation treatment', without understanding the fact that the abilities of these employees and their autism are inextricably linked.

This may sound fanciful but like other disability rights groups, those concerned with autism are keen to argue for the right to life and rightly oppose the possibility of abortion on the grounds of autism. Elizabeth Moon makes no secret of the fact that she has a son with autism and this experience clearly shows in her novel, both in terms of the creation of Lou but also in her value for those with autism. Currently, the argument about whether we should 'cure' autism is hypothetical, but it will only be a matter of time before genetic advances mean that it becomes a real possibility. I believe that the autism literature allows us a glimpse into the autistic world, in all its alien glory. We can shrink away from it or relish the multiplicity of viewpoints that it offers.

Both fictional and autobiographical accounts can help us to start to understand the autistic experience and empathise with those affected and their families. They also give us an insight into our own and society's attitudes towards autism. Through the previous examples I have illustrated the evolution of Western society's relationship with the condition. From taking peripheral parts in the narrative, people on the autistic spectrum now command their own storylines. They are revealed as fellow humans, albeit those with a fundamentally different way of understanding the world. Sometimes that way of understanding is shown not just as different but in a positive light. Sometimes the autistic world view is even shown as superior. This represents a massive change in societal attitudes.

References

Asperger, H. (1944) Die 'Autistischen Psychopathen' im Kindesalter. *Archiv für Psychiatrie und Nervenkrankheiten*, **117**, 76–136.

Asperger, H. (1974) Formen des Autismus bei Kindern. *Deutsches Artzeblatt*, **14**, 4.

Attwood, T. (1998) *Asperger's Syndrome: A Guide for Parents and Professionals*. Jessica Kingsley Publications.

Baker, N. (1988) *The Mezzanine*. Reprinted 1990. Granta Books.

Cesaroni, L & Garber, M. (1991) Exploring the experience of autism through first hand accounts. *Journal of Autism and Developmental Disorders*, **21**, 303–313.

Fitzgerald, M. (2005) *The Genesis of Artistic Creativity: Asperger's Syndrome and the Arts*. Jessica Kingsley Publications.

Grandin, T. & Scariano, M. M. (1986) *Emergence: Labeled Autistic*. Arena Press.

Haddon, M. (2003) *The Curious Incident of the Dog in the Night-Time*. Jonathan Cape.

Joyce, J. (1922) *Ulysses*. Reprinted 2000. Penguin Books.

Kanner, L (1943) Autistic disturbances of affective contact. *The Nervous Child*, **2**, 217.

Lee, H. (1960) *To Kill a Mocking Bird*. Heinemann.

Melville, H. (1853) *Bartleby, The Scrivener: A Story of Wall Street*. Reprinted (1990) as *Bartleby and Benito Cereno*. Dover Publications.

Toole, J. K. (1980) *A Confederacy of Dunces*. Reprinted 2006. Penguin Books.

Wing, L & Attwood, A. (1987) Syndromes of autism and atypical development. In *Handbook of Autism and Pervasive Developmental Disorder* (eds D. Cohen & A. Donnellan). John Wiley & Sons.

Index

Compiled by Caroline Sheard